Health Crisis, Counteractions and the Media in the Ibero-American World

Javier Jurado, Marina Ruiz Cano (eds.)

Health Crisis, Counteractions and the Media in the Ibero-American World

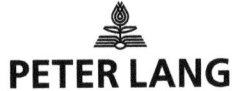

Lausanne - Bruxelles - Berlin - Chennai - New York - Oxford

Bibliographic information published by
the Deutsche Nationalbibliothek.
The German National Library lists this publication in the
German National Bibliography; detailed bibliographic data
is available on the Internet at http://dnb.d-nb.de.

Library of Congress Cataloging-in-Publication Data
A CIP catalog record for this book has been applied for at the
Library of Congress.

Cover illustration: © Javier Jurado

Published with support of Univ. Lille, ULR 4074 –
CECILLE - Centre d'Études en Civilisations, Langues
et Lettres Étrangères, F-59000 Lille, France.

ISBN 978-2-87574-872-0 (Print)
E-ISBN 978-2-87574-873-7 (E-PDF)
E-ISBN 978-2-87574-874-4 (E-PUB)
DOI 10.3726/b20803
D/2023/5678/67

© 2023 Peter Lang Group AG, Lausanne
Published by Peter Lang Editions Scientifiques Internationales - P.I.E.,
Brussels, Belgium

info@peterlang.com - www.peterlang.com

All rights reserved.
All parts of this publication are protected by copyright. Any
utilization outside the strict limits of the copyright law, without the
permission of the publisher, is forbidden and liable to prosecution.
This applies in particular to reproductions, translations, microfilming,
and storage and processing in electronic retrieval systems.
This publication has been peer-reviewed.

Table of contents

Introduction 9

Technical utopia and health dystopia: A contemporary visual battle 13
JAVIER JURADO

From the 1918 flu to Covid-19: A perspective from the Spanish case 23
PAU FONT MASDEU

The 1918 Influenza pandemic and its impact in the work of Ramón del Valle-Inclán and Josep Pla 43
JAUME SILVESTRE LLINARES

"Tourism Yes, Tourism No": The impact of the Covid-19 pandemic on discourse about tourism in the Spanish press 63
DAGMAR VANDEBOSCH

The inhumanity of neoliberalism and of the far-right in the context of the Covid-19 pandemic in Brazil 87
CÉSAR BOLAÑO AND FABRÍCIO ZANGHELINI

Health crises in images: Possible approximations between three major epidemics in Brazil 113
MARCELA BARBOSA LINS, CAIO DAYRELL SANTOS AND ÂNGELA CRISTINA SALGUEIRO MARQUES

Strategic communication and the vaccination plan of Covid-19: The Uruguayan case 137
   PATRICIA SCHROEDER

The challenge of higher education through virtual education platforms during Covid-19: The Peruvian case 171
   MARIANA NICOLINI ZEVALLOS AND GIANCARLO GOMERO

The July 11, 2021, protests in Cuba: A unique event? 193
   ORLANDO MANZANO GUERRERO

Epilogue: Intersectional solidarity and fairness in Ibero-American counteractions 221
   MARINA RUIZ CANO

Introduction

The health crisis resulting from the Covid-19 pandemic has irreversibly modified – and is still modifying – social, economic and cultural relations on a global scale, making this crisis an unprecedented event in the recent history of humanity. Covid-19 has clearly exposed social inequalities, which in Ibero-America have a particular character due to its socio-economic structure: the vast number of irregular jobs, the difficulties of accessing healthcare, the densification of urban spaces, etc. Although contagious and infectious diseases are undeniably a long-standing issue, the coronavirus epidemic has placed the world in an unprecedented health crisis, intensified by the characteristics of our societies, which is connected both geographically and in terms of communication.

Some of the consequences of this crisis are still today unforeseeable and to date have affected different social aspects such as tourism, education, cultural practices, working patterns, etc. Expert, political and lay actors publicly discuss the causes, developments and consequences of the epidemic, generating discourses on what is understood by pandemic, crisis, epidemic, etc. From the point of view of various disciplines from the human and social sciences, this volume questions the social effects of the pandemic in the Ibero-American world and proposes a discussion that allows us to put into perspective the antecedents, causes, synergies and consequences of this and other health crises.

The emergence and legitimisation of the modern state, and its coercive capacities, frame this reflection, which also aims to project itself into the more recent past (AIDS, syphilis, Spanish flu, etc.), not excluding the first years of the establishment of the nation-state, which, according to Foucault, established the biopolitical regime characteristic of contemporaneity.

Authors in this volume ask ourselves, then, what are the collective responses to the readjustments in social control imposed by the pandemic and in what way are they ascribed to political contexts (in the case of the Spanish ultra-right or the mobilisation for a new constitution in Chile), economic (the ebb and flow of so-called "tourism-phobia") or cultural (the subversive potential of confined theatre or the expansion of Netflix, HBO, Amazon Prime or Movistar).

In short, we propose a reflection on the socio-economic changes provoked or arising from this and other health crises, as well as the scope of cultural creation when it comes to answering, integrating or modifying the medical-political discourse of government bodies in Latin America and Spain.

These contributions are the result of an international congress that reunited researchers from different Latin-American countries interested both in Medical Humanities and Media Studies in a fruitful exchange that inspired this publication.

From a historical perspective, Pau Font Masdeu compares the discourses around the epidemics of 1918 and 2020 in Spain, rising the parallelisms as well as the inspiration academics the media took from the so-called "Spanish Flu".

This dialogue is also the matter of Jaume Silvestre's study around the works of Josep Pla et Ramón María del Valle Inclán during those last years of the 1910s decade. The interest Covid raised on how societies adapted to previous health crises had also found in literature a fertile ground for innovative research. Fever, delirium and creativity drive here a dialogue between these two writers which were both infected by the flu at the same time in two very different vital moments. But both are seminal figures of the *Silver age* of Spanish culture that developed in the first third of the 20th century.

Teacher Dagmar Vandebosch relies pharmaceutical and cultural industries with another key sphere of our modern economies that was most violently shaken by the Covid crisis. Tourism suffered a tremendous blow with travel restrictions all around the world, and in this article Vandebosch focalizes in Spain as well. In a country where tourism is frequently identified with European integration and economic development, discourses around freedom of movement became highly polarised and politicised. The opposition of Madrid's astronomical president, right-wing populist Isabel Diaz Ayuso, to the socialist government in almost every ground found in tourism a fertile ground to oppose libertarian freedom to "authoritarian State communism" as she denounces during her mandate.

Similar outbursts can be found in Bolsonaro's speeches in Brazil, thoroughly studied in César Bolaño's and Fabrício Zanghelini's article. They unveil the highly rational motivations that drive these apparently eccentric attitudes from extreme-right leaders. Deepening of neoliberal policies lies behind populist discourses of the now-defeated president. The consequences of these policies are suffered by the most fragile part of the society as is also shown in Marcela Barbosa Lins, Caio Dayrell Santos and Ângela Cristina Salgueiro Marques contribution. These three researchers not only follow the visual discourses raised by the Covid pandemic but also compare it with the 1918's flu and the yellow fever outbreak of the late 19th century. A biopolitical analysis of images and particularly photography of these three health crises allow the reader to follow the developement of a technocratic discourse that hides sickness as it promotes the modernization of the country through its medical bodies.

Since media and communication, as we have seen, are essential to health management, the contribution of Uruguay's communication advisor to the ministry of public health, Patricia Schroeder completes the account of political communication that most of the contributors to this book deal with. The informational strategy followed by the Austral country, analysed and exposed here in first person, supposes an unvaluable practical support to our study in a context where social media and the internet in general became a key factor in political communication.

Following this path, Giancarlo Gomero and Mariana Nicolini Zevallos focus on another sphere conditioned by the pandemic: education. Although the continuity of the learning processes was one of the main challenges countries all around the world had to deal with, the means made available to teachers and students have depended on the technology companies outside (initially) the school world. In line with what has been said so far, we can suggest here the hypothesis that one of the bastions of the welfare state, beset by the wave of liberalisation and privatisation since the 1980s, is facing a new offensive – this time with technological and efficiency arguments, thanks to the Covid crisis.

It is precisely with a very particular case of governance that we close our journey around health crises in Ibero-America. We are speaking about Cuba and it is thanks to the contribution of Dr. Orlando Manzano that we can dive into the causes and consequences of the protests that shook the island in July 2021. Even though we deal here with a different model, always under scrutiny and ground for political disputes, what we can draw from this account is the similarity of the fed-upness expressed by the Cuban people with that of the rest of the antagonistic discourses provoked by the pandemic worldwide.

Thanks to the contribution of Marina Ruiz Cano, this short introduction to our volume is completed and enriched notably with a gender perspective, clearly missing from our discussion until this point.

I take this opportunity to thank her and our workmate Camila Pérez Lagos for the invaluable help provided during the whole process of coordinating, preparing and publishing this research project. It would not have been possible either without the collaboration of professors Nadia Lie, Elizabeth Amann, Patricia Novillo-Corvalán and my personal friend and colleague Dr. William Rowlandson. I would like to thank M. Stéphane Thys as well who allowed this project to be possible despite the precarious university status of the editor of this volume, something that is rare and quite unique in the French University system.

Therefore, I would like to dedicate this volume to all those university workers who have seen their working conditions degrade over the last few years as well as to all the young (and not so young) researchers who continue to be punished by the lack of resources and often also of empathy. To all of them we send a big hug of solidarity.

Javier Jurado, Lille september 2023

Technical utopia and health dystopia: A contemporary visual battle

JAVIER JURADO *(Université de Lille)*

The relationship between public health and communication is complex and shifting, including attitudes that flow between necessity, mistrust, opportunity and denial as has been evident in the recent Covid-19 pandemic. The media need a flow of news to justify their relevance and aim to sell their products to citizens and consumers of a given society or social group with which they share a cultural and linguistic context (Hesmondhalgh, 2002: 179). In the case of news related to public health, the role of the media is somewhat contradictory to that of a public service in which coordination with state institutions is essential and necessary.

Contradictory, we say, because despite the fact that public health policies are based on the very statute of service to citizens, it does not escape from a political-partisan use that determines the quality and type of information that society receives (Castells, 2009: 196–213). The recent crisis demonstrates this last point, and the different information and/or opinion battles around subjects as varied as the origin of the pandemic, its vectors of transmission, and the measures to contain it and, later, to mitigate it are only examples of such use.

Looking at the United States, we can recall the confrontation that President Trump had with several media outlets, notably with CNN, as a result of the solutions proposed by the New York magnate. This was not an isolated event, and the pandemic – or rather the discourse surrounding it – became a political weapon in different countries and contexts, wherever it is possible to speak of the existence of a "free" press that is independent of the powers of the state.

Indeed, in democratic regimes, since the end of the 18th century, the press has had the status of a "fourth estate" that has served as a counterweight to various more or less corrupt or dishonest governments. This quality does not prevent us from ignoring the dependence of the media on the public authorities at the legislative or economic level, among others. It is not in vain that the emergence of public opinion itself goes hand in hand with the construction of the modern state, with the industrialisation that makes reproducibility technically possible (to borrow Walter Benjamin's concept), and with the very idea of public health.

It is in this interdependence that we pose the problem of this article, inspired by a prism of political ecology, which aims to show, through several examples taken from Europe, and from Spain in particular, the limits and biases of the discourse on public health conveyed by the media in our contemporary societies. After all, it is the very concept of contemporaneity that we intend to recontextualise in the light of the power of a section of the population over public discourses, which we restrict here more or less to health communication.

The triad of communication, democracy and industry is used here to analyse cases such as the Spanish flu, industrial and/or nuclear accidents or the AIDS crisis, as well as, obviously, the recent COVID pandemic. In this way, we can already advance a hypothesis taken from Fressoz and which we reformulate here to affirm that economic progress and industrialisation, which have become discursive elements inherent to our contemporary world, require the media to conceal or euphemise the consequences for both human beings and the environment.

Indeed, as Professor Font Masdeu states in this volume, the COVID pandemic has rescued from the memory of historians and journalists, among others, the 1918 flu, news of which was first reported in the Spanish press. Forced by wartime censorship, the European media made no reference to this disease, which would be christened "Spanish flu" precisely because of this journalistic censorship. War priorities, both in terms of the morale of the population and the medical-industrial capacity of the combatants, did not allow alarmism to spread any further in years when the war seemed to be dragging on much longer than expected.

The belligerent countries – and not only – were equally concerned about the spread of popular discontent among their own populations and, above all, in revolutionary Russia. In a particularly tense year 1917 in the rearguard, the possibility of a large-scale health crisis could not but worry both politicians and French, British and German industrialists because of its potentially devastating effects on war economies. The importance of hygienist and imperialist ideology could not accept the presence of diseased bodies in a struggle for preponderance of mankind.

If the First World War has been taken as an example of the massive use of propaganda at the state level, it is also because the self-image that was given as well as that of the enemy had to be inscribed in the coordinates presented by the crisis of growth, of industrial competition that fuelled the warmongering of European societies. The change of gear that Hobsbawm identified in world capitalism (1989: 34) was accompanied by a worldwide competition for resources in which communication played a key role.

This first episode of the European world war, which Enzo Traverso (2007) circumscribes to the period between 1914 and 1945, demonstrates the media's capacity for persuasion, particularly in conditions of monopoly of information, as indeed occurred in the Spanish Civil War and the Second World War, in which the word from the 1622 encyclical takes on a dark tinge and ultimately serves to group together Stalinist totalitarianism and Nazism.

From the ashes of the Nazi regime's manipulation of information through the ministry directed by Goebbels, the intellectuals of the Frankfurt School coined the critical theories of mass culture that would impregnate a pessimistic and mechanistic vision of communication that would last a very long time. If Adorno and Horkeheimer warned against the manipulative capacity of the culture industry in the singular, it was because they saw the reuse of the techniques used in their native Germany during the 1930s by the American entertainment industry that was soon to spread all over the planet.

Critical theory today finds itself criticised precisely for this mechanicism and branded as simplistic as well as for not taking into account the ability of consumers-citizens-viewers to have an opinion on cultural and mass communication products. However, it is in itself a reductionism to dismiss a whole reflection on industrial society and the importance of organised destruction in the lack of a critical alternative, which is, to a large extent, the great contribution of these intellectuals, and in particular of Herbert Marcuse.

> At its most advanced stage, domination functions as administration, and in the overdeveloped areas of mass consumption, the administered life becomes the good life of the whole, in the defense of which the opposites are united. This is the pure form of domination. (Marcuse, 2007: 259)

The evident denunciation of technocracy as the only alternative is not very far from the reality of post-industrial societies as well: this intuition about the scarce critical capacity of the industrial-capitalist productive system seems to us sufficiently relevant not to confine it to serving as an example of old-fashioned thinking when it comes to analysing the cultural industries. The germ of ecological critique can be another example that highlights the relevance of critical reflection.

This is particularly fruitful if we approach the communication around industrial catastrophes, almost unanimously labelled as "accidents" that have more to do with a risk capitalism that also presents these events as external to production or in any case transitory or exceptional (Fressoz, 2012: 248). The very concept of "externality" expels one of the most serious consequences that the industrial apparatus inflicts on the environment and the population.

Examples of this relativisation of the priority given to economic profit over public health abound in recent history. What is interesting is to see how this innate reality of the current economic system uses a particular vocabulary that allows us to dissociate responsibility from the primacy of the interests of a minority of the population. In this way, we can speak of the scandal of breast prostheses in France at the beginning of the 21st century or of rapeseed oil in Spain at the end of the 20th century. The very categorisation as a scandal means that these events are treated as an exception with little or no relation to industrial capitalism itself.

An unoriginal hypothesis that we put forward here is that economic growth is at the service of a minority of the population, a capitalist bourgeoisie with enormous influence over the media. We are not discovering anything by stating that the relativisation of these "accidents" or the concealment of the health, food, social and environmental problems caused by economic growth and industrial society is the norm in today's communication policy. And yet to hear a voice discordant with the ideology (prophecy) of continuous and ongoing progress is increasingly difficult in the state and/or international media.

The scale of the media, therefore, conditions the content and scope of the message, in a communicational ecology that is increasingly interconnected and in which large multinational companies occupy larger and larger market shares. The liberalisation and internationalisation of financial flows characteristic of the 1980s, as a consequence of the conservative revolution, produced the paradox of weakening the old state information monopolies, while the new actors – which were to serve as a counterpoint to official information – ended up converging with the former in terms of both information strategies and content (Bouquillion, 2008: 170).

Indeed, the internationalisation of information flows has given a power that would have been unimaginable a few years ago to communication actors such as News Corporation, Lagardère or Telefónica, to limit ourselves to the European information and communication market. This is the result of a global economic movement which is also reflected in an acceleration of trade and, as we have recently witnessed in a dramatic way, of the extent of health crises such as that of Covid.

In this sense, we share Benjamin Coriat's theory according to which the extractivism that dominates the economic logic of our current societies is at the heart of two major evils of what is also known as the anthropocene: climate change and the spread of zoonoses. To these two we add a third perverse effect that puts the very health of individuals at the centre through the processes of consumption. Indeed, the production and consumption of food and/or substances absorbed by our bodies deserve to be studied in order to understand the extent of environmental degradation in our own bodies. What became known as the Green Revolution of the 1950s and 1960s, which managed to alleviate the problems of malnutrition in important parts of the world, while producing enormous economic benefits for the agri-food industry, also brought about a transcendental change in the quality of the food itself.

The defence of these economic interests was accompanied by the certainty that world protein consumption was increasing exponentially with the use of chemical fertilisers and agro-fertilisers, which, however, also pose a risk to the food security of large groups of the population. Since the last third of the 20th century, food security has therefore been at the centre of public debate, but not without significant difficulties in reaching the media to establish a public debate on the effects on health, the environment and land ownership regimes. The best-known example of these efforts to make visible the aggressiveness of the methods and implementation strategies of the global agri-food industry was the Zapatista uprisings of peasants in the Chiapas region, directly affected by monoculture, the use of pesticides and fertilisers derived from petroleum and the commodification of raw materials included in the Free Trade Agreement (Soriano González, 2012).

Since the turn of the century, debates on public health (and in this case, food safety) have been imposed on the media agenda, in many cases, more as an advertising lure to get more audiences – due to a generalisation of sensationalism and enternews, to which the global Murdoch empire is no stranger – than as a scientific, economic or ecological debate. With the recomposition of the economy after the 1970s crisis and the general liberalisation of markets, few spheres of human activity remain outside the commodification imposed by the state and finance.

Public health is not left out of it. It is, in fact, one of the pillars of the welfare state that has been beset by the wave of deregulation following the conservative revolution of the 1980s. In some cases, these policies had the complicity of various centre-left governments, such as that of Felipe González in Spain or Mitterrand's policy of "reform brackets" (Carrey, 2017).

It is, however, in these years of global transformation of the economy that we can also situate one of the first health crises to arise with the liberalisation and internationalisation of markets, i.e., the heroin consumption crisis in Western Europe that devastated the youth of countries such as Spain in years when political freedom accompanied a youthful and utopian impulse known as the counterculture. The fact is that the lack of information and risk prevention policies resulted in the multiplication of deaths due to overdoses and AIDS infections, one of the great pandemics of the 20th century, which hit Western youth hard.

The atmosphere of liberalisation and liberalisation of the economy and information flows did not serve to warn of the risks of opiate use. Thus, in the face of growing political discontent – disenchantment, as it was called in Spain – with post-May '68 society, it was not channelled towards an alternative project that was collapsing with the end of the socialist bloc but rather drifted towards a hedonism that heroin also capitalised on, deepening not only depoliticisation but also a characteristic political and social apathy.

Even so, warnings about the advance of acquired immunodeficiency syndrome were heard by the homosexual population, which forced both governments to implement preventive measures and the media to make visible the ravages that this epidemic was causing. This is the case of Act-up Paris, which for months denounced the lack of information (Favereau, 2006: 74) that forced Jacques Chirac's government to declare AIDS a "national cause".

The other major group affected by this first major opiate crisis, namely drug addicts and the prison population, received less attention from the authorities and certainly less attention from the media. While awareness campaigns were late and focused on the young population, prevention and information policies for prisoners were practically non-existent (Tarrío, 1997). The situation of marginalisation and neglect in which the prisoners found themselves led to their mobilisation, both organisationally and through actions that would attract the attention of society and the media.

The 1990s marked a turning point in public health management, as Olivier Doubre (2020) explains, with the pharmaceutical and chemical industry emerging as a concurrent actor with institutional action on the one hand and patients themselves on the other. The relationship of forces between these three poles conditions the evolution of a new *bioeconomy* that is being established at the global level. The AIDS epidemic was the first major proof that the health threats to come were no longer localised, individual and manageable by the state but were becoming potential pandemics with effects on an increasingly mobile and globalised population, in which coordination between state and supra-state structures was becoming indispensable.

The recent Covid pandemic only confirms this premonitory hypothesis in which the media have become vectors of citizen accountability in the face of the state's ineffectiveness in controlling the flows of people and goods that have been increasing since the great liberalisation of the 1980s. Indeed, television has become the major government information agent for the years 2020 and 2021, for which communication teams have been set up to work alongside the private media, thus delegating a large part of the responsibility for health communication.

It goes without saying that the dependence of private actors on advertising funding and large industries (pharmaceutical and others) led to the generalisation of a discourse that was not free of sensationalism and created a social panic that concealed the economic origin of the zoonosis and the pandemic it caused. The main economic beneficiary of the so-called health catastrophes has been the pharmaceutical industry, as the management of vaccines has shamefully demonstrated.

The information and pharmaceutical industries are part of the same political and economic project based on the exploitation of both resources and the human and animal beings that populate the planet. This project is based on an extractivism that has been left out of any more or less reasonable and reasoned criticism in the mass media, exposing their interdependence with what we have called a global *bioeconomy* that escapes the control of states.

Thus, the accelerated industrialisation processes of the early 20th century that we mentioned at the beginning of the chapter were followed by the consolidation of business groups at the food, chemical and medical levels which, with the arrival of the great deregulation led by Reagan, Thatcher, and also by a new kind of socio-liberalism, achieved eloquent power and implantation at the supra-state level. The extractivist philosophy they advocate, which lies behind the great dangers that beset our times, is rarely mentioned in the media. Its effects: climate change and the multiplication of epidemics are presented in this way, disconnected from their conditions of production and reproduction, leaving a society at the mercy of interests that are not those of the majority of the population.

Bibliography

Bouquillion, Philippe (2008). *Les industries de la culture et de la communication. Les stratégies du capitalisme.* Grenoble: PUG.

Carrey, Claude (2017). "Une histoire politique de la France post-68". Unpublished.

Castells, Manuel (2009). *Communication Power.* Oxford: Oxford University Press.

Coriat, Benjamin (2020). *La pandémie, l'anthropocène et le bien commun.* Mayenne: Les Liens qui Libèrent.

D'Almeida, Fabrice (1995). *Images et Propagande.* Firenze: Casterman.

Doubre, Olivier (2020). "Vie / Mort", in *Une histoire (critique) des années 1990*, François Cusset (coord.), Paris: La Découverte.

Favereau, Éric (2006). *Nos années sida. 25 ans de guerres intimes.* Paris: La Découverte.

Fressoz, Jean-Baptiste (2012). *L'apocalypse joyeuse. Une histoire du risque technologique.* Paris: Seuil.

Hesmondhalgh, David (2002). *The Cultural Industries.* London: Sage.

Hobsbawm, Eric (1989). *The Age of Empire.* New York: Vintage Books.

Marcuse, Herbert (2007). *One-Dimensional Man.* London and New York: Routledge & Kegan Paul, 1964.

Soriano González, María Luisa (2012), "La configuración histórica e ideológica del zapatismo", *Anales de la Cátedra Francisco Suárez*, n. 46, pp. 237-257.

Tarrío, Xosé (1997). *Huye hombre, huye. Diario de un preso FIES.* Barcelona: Virus.

Traverso, Enzo (2007). *À Feu et à sang : De la guerre civile européenne, 1914–1945.* Paris: Stock.

From the 1918 flu to Covid-19: A perspective from the Spanish case[1]

PAU FONT MASDEU – *Universitat de Girona*

Introduction

The influenza pandemic of 1918–1919, better known as the "Spanish Flu", is considered the most important pandemic of the 20th century, with enormous demographic and economic consequences around the world. The most recent mortality studies estimate that it caused between 50 and 100 million deaths worldwide (Johnson & Mueller, 2002) and at least a third of the world's population became infected. In comparison, the flu killed more people than the Great War.

The epidemic unfolded in three waves, which occurred in the spring and autumn of 1918 and the beginning of 1919, with some variations in different continents. There are also some studies pointing to a brief fourth wave occurring in the first months of 1920. While the first and third waves were remarkably benign, with common flu symptoms and few complications, the second wave of the pandemic was global and with a high mortality rate due to pulmonary complications. In this regard, the regions with the highest mortality rates were Asia and Africa (with the highest rates up to 6 and 9 percent), whereas the pandemic had a lesser impact in Europe and North America. In Spain, the mortality rate is estimated at 1.2 percent, not far away from the 2.5 percent estimated worldwide rate (Spinney, 2017: 9). In contrast to other similar flu epidemics, the most affected age group was the young adult population, from 20 to 45 years (Taubenberger and Morens, 2006).[2]

---

[1] This text is part of the project "De la gripe de 1918 a la COVID-19: un análisis histórico en Europa y América Latina" de la Universitat de Girona, funded by the Fundación BBVA.

[2] This might be due to partial immunity acquired by the elderly population in past epidemics, like the 1889 "Russian" flu epidemic.

The debates on the origins of the virus are still active. The most remarkable studies point the focus to China or the United States (Phillips and Killingray, 2003), though there are also hypotheses that point to its origins in France due to the conjunction of soldiers, animals and chemicals during the Great War (Oxford et. al, 2005). Despite these debates, the War played a key role in the spreading (or even the emergence) of the pandemic, as "total war" mobilised large numbers of soldiers and workers around the world, often travelling in unhygienic and overcrowded conditions.

During the outbreak of the Covid-19 pandemic, attention was focused on the Spanish flu of 1918–19, due to the similarities between the two pandemics in health and sanitary terms. Many newspaper articles and television programmes (including sections on TV news) compared their similarities basically in terms of the measures taken to prevent and control the disease: face masks, disinfections, isolation, closure of leisure facilities, etc. It also became clear how little was known about the 1918 influenza culturally speaking and how few references were available beyond health comparisons. In Catalonia and throughout Spain, the memory of the flu focused almost exclusively on the literary reference of Josep Pla. The Catalan writer started his famous dietary *El Quadern Gris* by commenting on the closure of the university in Barcelona in the following months. Most of the articles used the *Quadern* quotations as a base, almost exclusively, to compare the 1918 Flu with the uncertain scenario at that time of 2020. Very few other authors or works were taken, neither from the same epidemic nor from other epidemics (except the plague and *The Decameron*).

This lack of references is closely related to the short-term memory of the 1918–19 influenza itself: there are no major traces of the epidemic beyond the years in which it lasted, let alone beyond the 1920s. This lack of memory (or memories) seems to be global, considering what Myron Echenberg (2003:238) explains in the case of Senegal, where the country's collective memory was centred on the memory of the endemic plague, despite the severity of the 1918 Flu. No process of constructing an official memory of the pandemic took place after 1919, largely due to the great impact of the Great War and its enormous consequences worldwide. Because of all of this, the Flu memory is neither direct nor explicit; it becomes swampy, and traces and connections in the following years are not clear.

As Covid-19 outbreak, the Spanish Flu took place in a complex political context. Through an approach based on political and cultural history, we can both answer questions related to the present and the past. This chapter, therefore, aims to analyse the relationship between the epidemic, politics and culture and to link these connections with the current situation produced by Covid-19.

Studying the Spanish Flu from a political and cultural perspective

The point that we wish to highlight is the direct relationship between the influenza pandemic and politics and culture, as mentioned above. Reviewing the existing literature, few works have focused on this aspect, and even fewer from the perspective of political and cultural history. At the same time, the absence of influenza in the historiographical production focusing specifically on the politics of the post-war years is even greater. This omission, which now seems glaring to us, has a reason: first, as already mentioned, the absence of short-term memory regarding the epidemic left few direct traces, few clear references to focus on. Moreover, studies on the estimation of deaths during the period 1918–19 have only recently been updated. We have only been aware of the huge demographic impact of influenza for a few years now. During the years following the epidemic, 21.5 million deaths were estimated (Jordan, 1927). By the 1990s, the figure had risen to 30 million (Patterson and Pyle, 1991), still far short of current estimates of 50 to 100 million. In turn, the significance of the Great War, its enormous consequences and the political and social analysis of the intense years that followed have also contributed to the influenza epidemic being overlooked. Political instability, demographic and economic imbalances and social unrest have always been associated with the direct effects of the global conflagration.

This is not to say that there are no useful studies for our analysis, nor do we intend to extensively review the previous literature. To begin with, the many studies that have contributed to understanding the disease from a medical, epidemiological or demographic point of view should not be underestimated. Such studies have been carried out from the years following the epidemic to the present day, as González García (2013) has pointed out.[3] Social history has also played an important role, relating this epidemic (and epidemics and diseases in general) to the social context in which they develop. In a combination of medicine, politics and social history, some of the first works with a deeper interpretation of the 1918 flu were produced. Moreover, the proliferation of numerous local and regional studies, with the incorporation of testimonies and experiences (Collier, 1974), has also contributed to offering a richer view of the epidemic as a global phenomenon.

With the adoption of new perspectives and the qualitative use of diverse sources, several works have appeared in recent years, close to the approach we are interested in. These collective books establish clear links between epidemics and culture, thus being good direct precedents for the approach we want to develop. Among them, the works coordinated by Howard Phillips and David Killingray (2003), or Ryan Davis and María Isabel Porras Gallo (2013) stand out.

The state of art for the Spanish case is similar to other European countries and the rest of the world. There are excellent overviews by Beatriz Echeverri (1993) and María Isabel Porras Gallo (2021),[4] which analyse beyond the strict health and medical aspects, paying attention to a significant extent to the social and political dynamics of the Spanish context. At the same time, it is worth mentioning a monograph by Ryan Davis (2013) on identity narratives in Spain during the epidemic, in which he highlights the link between the flu and the discursive narratives of the problems of Spain as a nation. On the other hand, there are also other works focused on the local or territorial aspects, which provide in-depth factual knowledge of the epidemic.

As mentioned, the links between epidemics and politics have not been widely explored, and, in consequence, the Spanish Flu is hardly related in the context of the post-war European period. We find one exception, precisely on the Spanish case, in an article by Blacik (2014) which links the 1918 epidemic with the political context 1917–1923 and connects it with the crisis of the Spanish political system and the beginnings of

---

[3] With no intention to provide an exhaustive list of works of this nature, we refer to this chapter.

[4] This book is a revised and substantially expanded version of the Ph.D. thesis *Un reto para la sociedad madrileña: la epidemia de gripe de 1918–19* (Universidad Complutense de Madrid, 1997).

Primo de Rivera's dictatorship. This example demonstrates the functionality of our approach.

Therefore, studying the Spanish Flu in Spain from a political and cultural perspective appears to be potentially fruitful. The Spanish context of this period is key to understand political and social evolution of the following years. Social unrest and political instability during that period led to the establishment of Primo de Rivera's dictatorship in 1923, set in a European context of democracy crisis and the rising of political authoritarian and antidemocratic alternatives and regimes. In addition, unlike other belligerent countries, in Spain we can rely on the press as a good source for analysing the harshest epidemic months, because of the lack of censorship that existed in countries at war that makes more difficult the epidemic's knowledge. Thus, the Spanish press becomes a great scenario to analyse information, debates and conflicts during the epidemic and its aftermath.

At this point, it is relevant to recall on Charles E. Rosenberg (1992:279) words. According to him, epidemics "constitute a transverse section through society, reflecting in that cross-sectional perspective a particular configuration of institutional forms and cultural assumptions". The Spanish Flu is not an exception. In this space, social, political and cultural dysfunctions emerge in both "material" and "discursive" ways. The "material" domain comprises the dysfunctions directly resulting from the epidemic, mainly concerns and criticisms of the government and health measures. As we will see, these material dysfunctions transcend the epidemic to, through it, expose debates about politics and society in a broad sense. In turn, during the epidemic months, a discursive association between epidemic and "evil" occurs. All the levers of conflict are permeated by an "epidemic language". The "evil" is present in every element of political discord and conflict: bolshevism, separatism, foreigners, etc.

Looking at the 1918–19 influenza pandemic from the present of Covid-19, a wide range of questions are now open to us, through which we can access our knowledge of the 1918 epidemic to find those elements that will also help us to ask questions about our present-day society. Ultimately, analysing politics and society through the epidemic will provide us new answers (and questions) about the period, opening up new perspectives and approaches.

The epidemic in Spain: Measures and responses

The influenza epidemic arrived in Spain in an extremely complex context. Although it did not take part in the war, Spain suffered acutely from its economic, social and political consequences since August 1914 (Fuentes Codera, 2021). The economic situation resulting from the war had led to a shortage of foodstuffs that considerably weakened the population, as well as an uncontrollable rise in prices. The months before the arrival of the pandemic were marked by the crisis of 1917, the impact of bolshevism derived from the Russian Revolution, social unrest, nationalist conflicts within the state (particularly Catalan nationalism) and the conflictive scenario in Morocco. The year 1918 saw the largest number of workers' mobilisations during the period 1914–18 with riots and strikes across the country, especially in industrial regions in Catalonia and the Anadalusian countryside (Romero Salvadó, 2008).

The political regime of the monarchic restoration designed by conservative statesman Antonio Cánovas in 1874 (after the failure of the First Republic) had reached a critical phase by 1918. What some historians called the "organic crisis" of the system led to parliamentary and governmental criticism, which became more pronounced after the triple crisis of 1917 (Romero Salvadó and Smith, 2010). The impact of influenza and the situation in the following months worsened the situation to a critical point.

In a broader context, the public health system as we know it today did not exist and, far from being what it is today, it had few resources. There was no Ministry of Health. Rather, public health system was part of the Interior Ministry (*Ministerio de la Gobernación*), which allocated derisory budgetary funds to health. The system was ruled by the old General Health Act (*Ley General de Sanidad*) of 1855, which was last amended in 1904 in the form of a regulation that did not meet the requirements of modern society (Porras Gallo, 2020:65). The situation of doctors was also precarious, as being employed by municipal governments and had little autonomy from mayors, who controlled the local politics through bossism (*caciquismo*). There were also hardly any hospitals and the charitable welfare organisations – usually religious – played a decisive role in caring for the sick. Municipalities also had an important role in health and sanitation management, but with limited means. Despite some progress since the second half of the 19th century, hygiene and sanitation were still poor, particularly in urban working-class neighbourhoods. In

Barcelona, for example, there had already been an epidemic of typhus in 1914, a disease closely related to deficiencies in the cleanliness of drinking water. Other epidemics like cholera, smallpox, tuberculosis and plague were constantly attacking the population due to a lack of control, hygiene and deficiencies in food.

In this general situation the first wave of influenza arrived in Madrid in May 1918. That first wave was generally benign. Few cases resulted in death and most of those infected experienced symptoms of common flu. The emergence of influenza was of little concern to the authorities and public opinion. In fact, the flu was firstly dubbed with humorous names: "the three-day fever", "the cockroach" (*La Cucaracha*) or the most popular one: "The Soldier of Naples" (*El Soldado de Nápoles*) after a song from *La Canción del olvido*, a famous *zarzuela* with a tune as catchy as the flu. Nonetheless, outside Spain, the influenza was called the "Spanish Flu" for one simple reason: Spain was the first country to officially report the epidemic because military censorship in the belligerent countries of the First World War covered up the presence of influenza.

It was during the second wave, in autumn 1918, that the epidemic began to have catastrophic consequences throughout the country. This wave was brought to Spain by travellers coming from France and travelled south across the country. Spanish workers, summer holidaymakers and Portuguese soldiers returning from the Western Front acted as involuntary spreaders of the epidemic (Porras Gallo, 2020:77). During the second wave, the virus caused more severe symptoms deaths. The first cases were detected in mid-August 1918, and the wave lasted until late November. The number of cases and deaths peaked in mid-October, coinciding with the final weeks of the war. Morbidity was high and the mortality rate in 1918 increased 50 per cent compared to the previous year. About 270,000 people died in Spain in 1918, which is the largest negative annual natural population growth rate since 1800 (Echeverri Dávila, 2003). In most of the country, the second and third waves overlapped in late autumn and early 1919.

At the end of September 1918, concerns and discussions about the health situation were close to those we saw in Spain by the beginnings of March 2020. The Spanish press, government and political parties began to take interest in the epidemic, with voices calling for more measures and others calling for less alarm in the face of a not-very-serious situation that was occurring. Authorities at both the central and provincial levels urged people to remain calm, speaking about a few cases and "well-prepared health services" across the nation.[5] Some measures were taken to prevent the spread of the epidemic, especially in border areas. In strategic points like rail stations and ports, health stations were set to increase controls at the border, disinfect passengers, perform medical exams and isolate sick people.[6]

After some days, when the epidemic grew significantly, some newspapers began to show concerns and measures spread everywhere. Crowding in enclosed spaces was prohibited and universities and schools were closed, as were bars and other leisure establishments. It was recommended to isolate the sick and that homes be well cleaned. The most common measure was spraying streets, public transport and passengers with disinfectant. Although many scientists advised that such disinfection was useless – because flu was spread from person to person though the air – these practices continued throughout the epidemic. With the current pandemic, we have also seen this type of useless action: tractors with tanks full of chemicals fumigating streets, the Military Emergencies Unit (*Unidad Militar de Emergencias*, UME) of the army disinfecting airports and train stations or, almost two years later and knowing fully well the transmission channels of Covid-19, members of the municipal brigade of the city of Badalona (the fourth largest city in Catalonia) spraying the surroundings of a primary health centre with bleach.[7]

In 1918 there were no such harsh measures as lockdown, but compliance with the measures was limited and far from uniform. As the press reported constantly, the public had little awareness and education on hygiene and health issues. While the establishments were closed, festivities and religious events continued to be held throughout the country, acting as hotspots for the spread of the disease. A notorious case reported by Spinney (2017:82–5) exemplifies it: in the city of Zamora, nine days of prayers were organised with also a crowded procession to protect the population from the disease. The city, far from being saved, had one of the highest mortality rates in the whole country at the end of the second epidemic wave. In a same way, the provincial health inspector of Valladolid explained in his memoirs of the epidemic the situation he

---

[5] Pérez, Darío (1918, September 14), "Desde San Sebastián. La cuestión sanitaria", *Heraldo de Madrid*.

[6] (1918, September 14), "Medidas sanitarias", *La Vanguardia*.

[7] (2021, December 23) "Badalona desinfecta els carrers per on passa més gent contra el COVID", *Ara*.

encountered when visiting a village struck by the disease (García Durán, 1920:19):

> Our impression on the arrival in this town could not have been more painful: the bells were ringing for the dead, the streets were deserted, and in contrast to this picture, as we crossed the Plaza Mayor, where the Town Hall is located, a palisade of thick timber bore witness to the fact that not many days before a feast of young bulls [*fiesta de novillos*] had been held there. In a full epidemic state, with some seriously ill in most of the houses, with many families already in mourning for the deaths that had occurred… Can there be any greater proof of the degree of a people's ignorance about health?

In contrast to this compliance with measures and recommendations within the country, the zeal to prevent the entry of the disease from the outside stood out. As we have seen in today's far-right politicians with Covid-19, the "foreign enemy", has been blamed for bringing the virus within the borders of the territory. In 1918–19, the stigma and accusations of the "other" bringing the virus, when the virus was already rampant throughout Spain, were constant. In already existing calls for the closure of the border, particular blame was directed at Portuguese soldiers returning from war who had to cross Spain to return home. Several examples are found in the press, demanding measures to avoid the entry of foreigners to "free Spain from the horrors of an epidemic imported from France by Portuguese soldiers".[8] The government focused their efforts in controlling the borders, limiting the entry to Spaniards, who were required to undergo a medical examination before entering the country. The main border health stations at Irún and Portbou, as well as the one at Medina del Campo (an important railway hub), were subjected to severe pressure from the local population and the opinion of the press. The installation of beds for the sick, disinfections and medical examinations was considered essential to stop influenza.

Despite the measures taken in sanitary border stations, alarm grew among the population and the press due to the lack of control. There were constantly rumours and reports of irregular entry of people across the border, and the authorities were heavily criticised. This situation went beyond the worst months of the epidemic. In May 1919, the villagers of Torrevieja, in Alicante province, "rioted to prevent the disembarkation" of a Norwegian vessel with twelve sick sailors on board. Fear of contagion

---

[8] (1918, October 29), "El estado actual de la epidemia. La salud Pública", *La Acción*.

and memory of the severe outbreak of autumn 1918 kept people on the alert, which sometimes led to violent situations. In Santa Cruz de Tenerife even in February 1920, "a large number of local residents, led by the parish priest brandishing a revolver, objected to the disembarkation" of a vessel with sick people on board.[9]

Overall, the consequences of the epidemic were extremely harsh, especially during the second wave from September to November 1918. The lack of medicines and doctors were constant. Sickness and death overtook towns and cities, as health care and funeral services were stretched to the limit. This was particularly true in Barcelona during October 1918, when there was a shortage of coffins and carts to carry the dead (Rodríguez Ocaña, 1991: 147). The press strongly denounced this situation, which was impossible for the authorities to resolve.

Although influenza affected the whole society (even the King Alfonso XIII fell sick), it affected particularly hard the poorer strata of society. The behaviour of the epidemic in this respect is comparable to that experienced with Covid-19. All epidemics strike everyone, but it is the poorest people who experience the misery and the worst consequences. In 1918, the poor were also blamed for the spread of contagion. Overcrowding and poor hygienic conditions in poor neighbourhoods were seen as infection hotspots by the authorities. The most extreme case of this blame occurred in Alicante, as Pascual Artiaga (2014) exposes. The barrack neighbourhood *Las Provincias* was entirely demolished for being considered the focus of the epidemic in the city. Families who lived there were forced to move to other parts of the province and the country. During the current pandemic, situations in these kinds of informal settlements have been also harsh and the focus has also remained on their sanitation conditions. Indeed, the UN-Habitat developed a programme not only to coordinate, inform, map out and mitigate the effects of Covid-19 in informal settlements, particularly in poor countries, but also to provide "structural solutions to the very problems which render them so vulnerable".[10]

Going back to 1918, ultimately, the measures taken to stop the epidemic waves were completely insufficient. The entire political spectrum,

---

[9] (1920, February 18) "El miedo a la gripe. Centenares de disparos contra el vapor 'Fuerteventura'", *El Sol*.

[10] United Nations – Habitat (2022), *UN-Habitat's COVID-19 Response Plan*. URL: https://unhabitat.org/un-habitat-covid-19-response-plan

as well as the opinion expressed in the press, saw the inefficiency of the State as the cause of the epidemic disaster. Lack of medical staff, medicines, disinfection equipment and foresight proved to be a problem related to the State dysfunctionality, from central government to local councils. The impact of the outbreak and criticism, far from being limited to the epidemic itself, went much further.

The aftermath: The "evil" and the criticism of the regime

As said before, epidemics are a cross-section of a society and a context. Beyond the criticisms generated strictly by the management of the epidemic, the flu was used as a weapon against political opponents, linking the contagion with the "evil". In both "material" and discursive ways, we find a great example in the Catalan region and the conflict between Catalan and Spanish nationalism. And also, then and in 2020.

Conservative Catalanism, represented by the Regionalist League (*Lliga Regionalista*) Party and its leader Francesc Cambó had been trying for years to achieve reforms of the political system in Spain and Catalonia. These aspirations clashed with the impossibility of achieving any democratising openness in favour of Catalan autonomy. With the end of the Great War and Wilson's speech recognising the rights of national minorities, the last attempt to grant Catalonia a Statute of Autonomy took place (Smith, 2010:151–2). These aspirations caused tension and raised the alarm among certain sectors of Spanish nationalism, seeing Catalan aspirations as a threat to the integrity of the State. Amid the outbreak in late 1918, the management of the epidemic was used to stoke the conflict.

During the harshest month of October, when Barcelona was suffering from a situation of sanitary overflow, the *Lliga*'s newspaper *La Veu de Catalunya* complained that some Madrid newspapers were exaggerating the situation in Barcelona,[11] while the conservative daily *ABC* of Madrid spoke of "abandonment" and of a management of the epidemic "as useless as the City Council".[12]

---

[11] (12/10/1918), "En defensa de la ciutat", *La Veu de Catalunya*.
[12] (1918, October 13), "Un caso inaudito de incúria y de abandono", *ABC*.

After the worst moments of the flu, the campaign for autonomy took off and reached the Spanish Congress. In an aggressive article, Dr José María Albiñana[13] called for a reminder of the lamentable example of Catalonia during the epidemic before granting any autonomy. He asked to "the new liberators of Catalonia": "In the name of what superiority do administrators who are not even capable of burying their own dead ask for autonomy?".[14] In a discursive way, Catalan nationalist were ridiculed by some newspapers. *La Acción* wrote: "Regionalist fever will cause more deaths than the flu".[15] From *El Globo* and in a sarcastic tone, it was said that autonomy was an epidemic produced by the bacillus *catalanis lliga*, being its producing agents a "portion of parasites and microbes".[16]

From the Catalan side, the epidemic was also used as a political argument. After attending a health rally in Madrid, the republican politician Àngel Samblancat stated that "epidemics are not extinguished with rallies" and that "Spanish politics is not the politics of life, but the politics of death".[17] These sentiments resonate strongly with many in Catalonia. In April 2020, regional MP Joan Canadell, from right-wing Catalan independentist party *Junts per Catalunya*, stated in a tweet addressed to the "Spaniards" that "independent Catalonia would have saved thousands of lives. (…) Spain is unemployment and death, Catalonia is life and future",[18] accusing the Spanish government of not having ordered earlier the lockdown in March 2020.

In flu-hit Spain of 1918–19, we also find this kind of metaphoric links in the disqualification of trade unionism and Bolshevism. The newspaper *La Acción* wrote about a "virus" and a "moral epidemic" referring to the rising strength of socialism.[19] In a same way, the journalist

---

[13] Neurologist. Influenced by Mussolini, in 1930 he founded the Spanish Nationalist Party (*Partido Nacionalista Español*), a monarchist and extreme right-wing party. He took part in general Sanjurjo failed military coup of 1932 and the Spanish coup of July 1936.
[14] Albiñana, José María (1918, December 12), "Aspecto sanitario. Del problema catalanista", *ABC*.
[15] El Bachiller Manzanares [pseudonym] (1918, December 1), "Siluetas de la semana", *El Globo*.
[16] F. de Viu [pseudonym] (1918, November 27), "¡Nos han regionalizado!", *La Acción*.
[17] Samblancat, Àngel (1918, December 11), "Política sanitaria", *El Diluvio*.
[18] (2020, April 22), "Canadell: 'Espanya és atur i mort, Catalunya és vida i futur'", *Nació Digital*.
[19] (1918, October 19), "Una epidemia moral", *La Acción*.

Carlos Rojas, ironized at the beginning of the outbreak how easy it was to combat a "mere flu", whereas "the bacteria of socialism (...) must be attacked with very costly specifics. We prefer the bacillus".[20] This is a sort of discursive parallelism that has been drawn in the current epidemic with VOX far-right Spanish political party leaders speaking of the danger of the "Chinese communist virus". According to them, a virus that must be fought with the strength of "the hands of the Spaniards".[21] Similar xenophobic words have come out of President Donald Trump's mouth and other far-right politicians across the world.[22]

Beyond all that, the neckbone that transcends the epidemic of 1918–19 in Spain itself is the criticism of the State and the political regime. As we have seen, measures set to stop the flu were insufficient and seen as a sign of the State's dysfunctionality. From the beginning of the second wave, criticism was aimed at the government. They were accused to act wrongly and too late. In a context of political instability, criticism of the political regime by the press and politicians across the ideological spectrum shook its foundations. Doctors, who played an important media role during the second wave, also blamed the State for the long-standing neglect of care services. Overall, politicians, intellectuals and professionals (in this case doctors, but also pharmacists and veterinarians) identified the influenza epidemic as another element that highlighted – and at the same time destabilised – the Restoration regime (Blacik, 2009:249).

Spanish intellectuals also assumed the influenza epidemic as another element of national decadence, in another discursive fusion of "evil" with the epidemic. The *regeneracionista* term "national disease" (in other words, the moral decadence of Spain) manifested itself through practical inefficiency and physical decadence, both produced by the influenza epidemic. As José Ortega Munilla wrote during the outbreak: "We must react against the mortal ailment that Spain is suffering, which is not this protean and disconcerting flu (...) it is the national disease."[23]

---

[20] Rojas, Carlos, "Los Hombres y los Días. El bacilo de Nápoles", *La Acción*, 26/05/1918.
[21] Ortega Smith, J. [@Ortega_Smith], (2021, April, 13), *Contra el virus comunista, la libertad y la unión de una nación soberana* [Tweet]. Twitter: https://twitter.com/orteg a_smith/status/1382064493283438599
[22] Rogers, Katie, Lara Jakes, and Ana Swanson (2021, March 18), "Trump Defends Using 'Chinese Virus' Label, Ignoring Growing Criticism", *The New York Times*.
[23] Ortega Munilla, José (1918, October 19), "Por los héroes de la epidemia", *La Nación*.

The need of regenerating the nation was shared by all the political forces. The question was how to do it. For many, the solution to the inefficiency of the state and the decadence of the nation laid in technocratic management by experts who would remove political incompetence from fundamental decisions. Ortega y Gasset, at the height of the second wave, suggested that "cultivated Spaniards" should take charge of the situation: "doctors, engineers, teachers, academics, artists, industrialists".[24] From November of 1918 to May 1920, there were as many as five successive governments, while antiliberal and antidemocratic ideas were gaining ground, from the left as well as the right. Strikes and social unrest completed the equation. The socialist intellectual Luis Araquistáin pointed the political situation: Spain was in a crossroads between "revolution" and "an antidemocratic and antiliberal dictatorship".[25]

From the beginnings of the epidemic, calls for a "health dictatorship" were made by politicians, intellectuals, doctors and the press. The idea was supported by the belief that an "expert" with hard hand and no political inferences could solve the nation's sanitary problems. The national decline had to be fought developing a modern and strong health system to avoid death. The Interior minister itself referred to "health dictatorship" while speaking about the measures adopted by the government.[26] In a same line, some of the press also supported the control of information in order to manage correctly the outbreak. These "health dictatorship" calls are clearly a mixture of criticism to government and politics inaction and the regenerationist "national disease", the decline of the nation, and show how authoritarianism would be welcomed as a form of government.

Towards dictatorship: Authoritarianism and democracy at stake

Calls for a "health dictatorship" continued beyond the pandemic. In 1921, Dr Martín Salazar, General Inspector of Health, still remarked the need for a "health dictatorship" to solve the inefficiency of sanitary

---

[24] Ortega y Gasset, José (1918, October 9), "Los Nuevos Gobiernos que necesita España", *El Sol*.

[25] Araquistáin, Luis (1918, November 7), "Entre dos dictaudras y una revolución", *España*.

[26] (1918, October, 2), "La cuestión sanitaria. Dictadura desde las esferas del gobierno", *Heraldo de Madrid*.

and health organization in the country.[27] In the political field, same calls remained as many came to see "health dictatorship" as the only solution. Antonio Maura reclaimed it, because "nowhere has this been remedied but by dictatorship".[28]

Despite these calls throughout the parliamentary spectrum, only the Right transcended the barrier of calling for a dictatorship *tout court*. Both "health dictatorship" and dictatorship started mixing in 1919, when social unrest and political destabilization started being acute. At the same time, as pointed by Victoria Blacik (2009:273), these connections link the appeals to the dictatorship with the flu epidemic, which had always been seen as having started in 1919.

Following the epidemic and the appeals to dictatorship due to the depletion of political regime, Miguel Primo de Rivera stated a coup d'état on 13 September 1923. As Alejandro Quiroga analysed accurately (Quiroga Fernández de Soto, 2007), the dictatorship used a scientific and medical language as a rhetorical element that keeps a close relation to the "health dictatorship". Indeed, a clear example is found in the coup itself. Primo de Rivera stated that his aim was to heal "the sick body of the nation" and eliminate the "cancer" of oligarchy (Blacik 2009: 273).

References to the flu during the dictatorship are not as clear as we have seen until now. But the directory put enormous efforts in improving the health and sanitary organization across the country with a new organization and legislation. Demands made by doctors during the epidemic were largely met. The Provincial Health Regulations, enacted in 1925, created Provincial Institutes of Hygiene led by provincial health inspectors. The following year, the Municipal Health Regulations created the Corps of Municipal Health Inspectors, who were to work independently of local authorities.

It is a fact that health improved in Spain during these years, something that was exploited by the regime's propaganda. Forward in 1927, it was remarked in the regime's official magazine *Unión Patriótica*, contrasting the effective labour of the current General Director of Health Dr Francisco Murillo: "Our rulers realised that the only effective policy is that which is based on defending health, saving the race and preparing

---

[27] (1921, June 9), "La Sanidad en el Estado", *España Médica*.
[28] (1921, June 4), "El señor Maura y la dictadura sanitaria", *La Acción*.

strong and vigorous generations." Dictatorship ended with the inefficient parliamentary system:

> The form of government that governs us has also avoided the excesses of parliamentarianism, the political diatribes and dilatory corruption to which the action of the *Cortes* were part, which always created difficulties and obstacles for health matters (…) The success of Dr. Murillo's work is a success that was foreseen and is the consequence of having brought to control the destinies of health, not an intriguer, nor a politician, nor an improvised person, nor a legislator, but simply a man of science.[29]

The dictatorship, led by experts, had saved the homeland from parliamentary ineptitude. No doubt, the epidemic context of 1918–19 and public policies carried out by the dictatorship, especially from 1925 onwards, keep a close continuity relation.

Focusing now again on the relation between epidemics and politics, parallelisms between the 1918–19 and the Covid-19 pandemic contexts are more than evident. The Europe of the Spanish flu was struggling to emerge from the aftermath of the Great War; the European context at the eruption of Covid-19 was still marked and conditioned by the profound changes brought about by the 2008 financial crisis. And now, in (what appears to be) the end of this pandemic, the economic damage of Putin's war in Ukraine, especially on the price of supplies and electricity, is added to the economic consequences of the pandemic. In turn, many of the arguments seen in the context of the flu epidemic and the following years also keep a close relation to the current situation like "health dictatorship" and call for an "expert" to solve the issues that politics can't manage. Also, some rhetoric analysed is used nowadays by the far-right movements.

The use of scientific and medical language as a rhetoric element is not new in politics. Blaming "the enemy" as a carrier of a virus is something we have seen not only in the 1918–19 context but also later in fascist regimes. The current pandemic has seen expressions of xenophobia and racism blaming the contagion on the "way of life of our immigrants"[30]

---

[29] Álvarez Sierra, J. (1927, November 1), "D. Francisco Murillo y Palacios", *Unión Patriótica*.

[30] This example is found in the words by Isabel Díaz Ayuso, President of Madrid Regional Government. Viejo, Manuel and Juan José Mateo (2020, September 15), "Ayuso señala que algunos contagios de Madrid se producen por el modo de vida de los inmigrantes", *El País*.

that use medical and allegedly scientific arguments to justify completely unscientific political positions.

Some voices have also called for the pandemic to be managed by experts, because of the distrust of politicians and politics. This disaffection always favours the backward sectors of society. Also, from citizens' movements backed by the new far-right movements, they have spoken out against restrictions and epidemic control measures, which they describe as a "health dictatorship" against personal liberty. The use of the term "health dictatorship" has different meanings in both contexts.

As Maximiliano Fuentes explained, today's far-right discourses "share an appeal to an idea of freedom based on a libertarianism with neoliberal roots that has little to do with the diatribes against liberalism and democracy of the right-wing of the first post-war period". But beyond that, and here is the central issue, they share "a critique of politics understood as an expression of democratic and parliamentary mechanisms".[31] Both yesterday and today's movements share the criticism to the "excess of politics". And what is in question is, at the end, liberal democracy. In the post-war context and in the 1920s, it was ended from outside the system; now, the aim is to erode it from within.

The twenties' authoritarian regimes and movements emerged from a post-pandemic context, even though they did not identify themselves as such. Today's (post) pandemic present continues to offer authoritarian and anti-democratic impulses. The dizzying pace of the present prevents us from analysing where we are with the right perspective. But from all the reflections raised, many of which offer a great deal of food for thought, we can derive the desire expressed at the beginning: trying to better understand our present in the light of the past. Beyond comparisons in health terms and from what it seems so far, our future still holds some more time of epidemics, of questioning democracy and, of course, of the relationship between one and the other.

Bibliography

Blacik, Victoria (2009). "De la desinfección al saneamiento: críticas al Estado español ldurante la epidemia de gripe de 1918", in *Ayer*, 75, 3, 247–273.

---

[31] Fuentes, Maximiliano (2021, December, 14), "Sobre la 'dictadura sanitaria'", *CTXT*.

Collier, Richard (1974). *The Plague of the Spanish Lady*. New York: Atheneum of Books for Young Readers.

Davis, Ryan (2013). *The Spanish Flu. Narrative and Cultural Identity in Spain, 1918*. New York: Palgrave Macmillan.

Echenberg, Myron (2003). "'The Dog That Did Not Bark'. Memory and the 1918 Influenza Epidemic in Senegal", in *The Spanish Influenza Pandemic of 1918–19: New Perspectives*, Howard Phillips and David Killingray (eds.), London: Routledge, 230–238.

Echeverri Dávila, Beatriz (2003). "Spanish Influenza Seen from Spain", in *The Spanish Influenza Pandemic of 1918–19: New Perspectives*, Howard Phillips and David Killingray (eds.), London: Routledge, 173–190.

——— (1993). *La Gripe Española. La pandemia de 1918–1919*. Madrid: Siglo XXI.

Fuentes Codera, Maximiliano (2021). *Spain and Argentina in the First World War. Transational Neutralities*, Abingdon: Routledge.

González García, Alberto (2013). "Avances y tendencias actuales en el estudio de la pandemia de gripe de 1918-1919", in *Vínculos de Historia*, 2, 309–330.

Johnson, Niall P.A.S, and Juergen Mueller, (2002). "Updating the Accounts: Mortality of the 1918–1920 'Spanish' Influenza Pandemic", in *Bulletin of the History of Medicine*, 76, 92–104.

Jordan, Edwin (1927). *Epidemic Influenza, a Survey*. Chicago: American Medical Association.

Oxford, John S., et. al. (2005). "A Hypothesis: The Conjunction of Soldiers, Gas, Pigs, Ducks, Geese and Horses in Northern France during the Great War Provided the Conditions for the Emergence of the 'Spanish' Influenza Pandemic of 1918–1919", in *Vaccine*, 23, 940–945.

Pascual Artiaga, Mercedes (2014). "Epidemic Disease, Local Government, and Social Control. The Example of the City of Alicante, Spain", in *The Spanish Influenza Pandemic of 1918–1919*, María Isabel Porras Gallo and Ryan Davis (eds.), Rochester: University of Rochester Press, 215–229.

Patterson, David K., and Gerald F. Pyle (1991). "The Geography and Mortality of the 1918 Influenza Pandemic", in *Bulletin of the History of Medicine*, 65, 4–21.

Phillips, Howard, and David Killingray (eds.) (2003). *The Spanish Influenza Pandemic of 1918–19: New Perspectives*. London: Routledge.

Porras Gallo, and María Isabel (2020). *La gripe española 1918–1919*. Madrid: Catarata.

────── and Ryan Davis (eds.) (2014). *The Spanish Influenza Pandemic of 1918–1919*. Rochester: University of Rochester Press.

Quiroga Fernández de Soto, Alejandro (2007). *Making Spaniards: Primo de Rivera and the Nationalization of the Masses, 1923–30*. New York: Palgrave Macmillan.

Rodríguez Ocaña, Esteban (1991). "La grip a Barcelona: un greu problema esporàdic de salut pública. Epidèmies de 1889–90 i 1918–19" in *Cent anys de salut pública a Barcelona*, Antoni M. Roca Rosell (coord.), Barcelona: Ajuntament de Barcelona, 131–156.

Romero Salvadó, Francisco J. (2008). *The Foundations of Civil War: Revolution, Social Conflict and Reaction in Liberal Spain, 1916–1923*. London: Routledge.

Rosenberg, Charles E. (1992). *Explaining Epidemics and Other Studies in the History of Medicine*. New York: Cambridge University Press.

Smith, Angel, (2010). The Lliga Regionalista, the Catalan Right and the Making of the Primo de Rivera Dictatorship, 1916–1923 in *The Agony of Spanish Liberalism: From Revolution to Dictatorship, 1913–23*, Francisco J. Romero Salvadó and Angel Smith, (eds.), Hampshire: Palgrave Macmillan.

Spinney, Laura (2017). *Pale Rider: The Spanish Flu of 1918 and How It Changed the World*. New York: PublicAffairs.

Taubenberger, Jeffery K. and David M. Morens (2006). "1918 Influenza: The Mother of All Pandemics", in *Emerging Infectious Diseases*, 12 (1), 15–22.

The 1918 Influenza pandemic and its impact in the work of Ramón del Valle-Inclán and Josep Pla

JAUME SILVESTRE LLINARES – *Open University of Catalonia*

The recent Covid-19 pandemic has brought to the fore the role of literature in conceiving the world and resituating our position in it, besides assessing its healing effect based on a certain worldview. The number of pages written about this pandemic is notorious, from essays, novels, compendiums, diaries to audio-visual works. In fact, the philosopher Slavoj Zizek reminds us of this intimate link between health and literature, since he considers that the Covid-19 pandemic is ironically explained in H. G. Wells's *The War of the Worlds* (1897), although in an inverted way, since it deals with "the story of how after Martians conquer the earth, the desperate hero-narrator discovers that all of them have been killed by an onslaught of earthly pathogens to which they had no immunity: "slain, after all man's devices had failed, by the humblest things that God, in his wisdom, has put upon this earth" (2020: 12).

This current context has entailed a diachronic view in order to show that literature has long been a clear prism to enter the world of health at critical moments in history. Epidemics, pandemics and diseases have been constantly reflected by writers, either because they have suffered from these conditions or because of literary interest. Let us briefly recall some examples, such as the *Decameron* (1349) by G. Boccaccio, *A Journal of the Plague Year* (1722) by Daniel Defoe, *The Mask of the Red Death* (1842) by E. A. Poe, *The Plague* (1947) by A. Camus, *Blindness* (1995) by J. Saramago or *L'estany de foc* (2010) by S. Vilaplana.[1]

---

[1] In addition, anthological publications that focus on literary texts that refer to diseases have been constant. We cite, for example, the work *Literatura i pandèmia. Antologia de texts* (2021), edited by Montserrat Camps. It should be added that in addition to this retrospective vision, there are also numerous literary works in many cultures that appeal to Covid-19 or pseudo-epidemics, such as *Un kilometro. Poesía e imágenes en la frontera* by Carmen Valencia and Paco González, the collective work *De los días*

Precisely, this research is part of this growing interest in what literature can teach us in relation to health. To do this, we have chosen two 20th-century prominent authors of Spanish and Catalan letters, whose trajectories were marked by another flu dating back a century ago, the one of 1918, an infectious disease with no cure at the time. They are Ramón María del Valle-Inclán (1866–1936) and Josep Pla (1897–1981), who were actually infected by this flu, the first during the second wave in October 1918 and the latter during the third in February 1919. At that time the age difference between them was considerable, the Galician writer was 52 years old, while the Catalan was 21, but there is evidence that they met and shared literary gatherings in Madrid in 1921, as confirmed by Pla in his work Madrid 1921. Un dietario "a ambos los conozco personalmente; a Azaña, de un café literario o de otros lugares, de los frecuentados por don Ramón del Valle-Inclán y su cuñado Rivas Cherif" (Pla 2020[1957]: 214).[2] Thus, we will investigate the impact of the aforementioned pandemic on two writers in two different vital moments: the Galician in the stage of consolidation of his work and the Catalan in his formative one.

Therefore, based on their works and their vital circumstances, we will explore the impact that this epidemic had on their literary careers, an aspect referred to by critics superficially. In this way, we will point out what analogies and divergences can be established in relation to the literary and personal effect of the same disease in his literary work, while we will try to assess certain topics or myths, as is the case of artistic prolificacy during confinement, and the written reflection of the pandemic in his works.

Valle-Inclán and the 1918 influenza pandemic

Undoubtedly, no introductions are necessary from Ramón María del Valle-Inclán, a well-known author of Hispanic letters, whose life and work has been analysed countlessly in articles, monographs, newspapers

---

[2] *sin abrazos. 25 obras en confinamiento*, Summer by Ali Smith or El Palomar by Tina Vallès.
In the same work, Pla again refers to Valle-Inclán to highlight his admiration and erudition "hay en Madrid unas cuantas personas admirablemente adiestradas. De Valle-Inclán, por ejemplo, todo el mundo os dice que es un hombre que tiene "una cultura muy rara". ¿Qué será eso -me pregunto yo?" (2020: 177).

or essays. This consideration could also be transferred to Josep Pla, who shared with him very similar tribulations marked by the history of the first half of the 20th century in Spain, Catalonia and Europe. However, in their wanderings across that Spain that was a political powder keg at that time, another more mundane but terribly fatal circumstance crossed their lives: health or lack of it. As we will see below, the 1918 flu marked both lives and literary careers.

Let's start by gleaning the impact of the 1918 influenza pandemic in Valle-Inclán. For this purpose, it is peremptory to refer to one of the most famous literary references in relation to this disease, recently echoed by society:

> Como hay tanta gripe, han tenido que clausurar la universidad. Desde entonces, mi hermano y yo vivimos en casa, en Palafrugell, con la familia. Somos dos estudiantes ociosos. A mi hermano, que es un gran aficionado a jugar al fútbol—a pesar de haberse roto ya un brazo y una pierna—lo veo solamente a las horas de comer. Él hace su vida. Yo voy tirando. No añoro Barcelona y menos aún la universidad. La vida de pueblo, con los amigos que tengo aquí, me gusta. (Pla 2016[1966]: 589)

Precisely, we have brought up the words of Pla, which represent one of the first literary references to the 1918 flu which, as we can see, supposedly forced the closure of educational centers from the spring of 1918. We refer to this quote due to the concomitance with the life of Valle-Inclán, who in June 1918 left Madrid to take refuge in the town of A Pobra do Caramiñal (Coruña). Thus, both preferred to confine themselves to the tranquillity of Palafrugell and A Pobra, far from the agglomerations of Barcelona and Madrid where Pla studied and Valle-Inclán worked. As we will see below, the Great Influenza epidemic had a decisive role in the literary production of the Galician author, since the one-year confinement was the period of his greatest artistic creation.

In this way and paradoxically, Valle-Inclán found in the calm of A Pobra the necessary inspiration to write tirelessly during a mournful historical period, thus promoting his literary career and succinctly improving the migrated state of his coffers. Let's analyse the ups and downs of his confinement in the pazo de la Merced between 1918 and 1919.

The biography of the author from Coruña shows us that his residence passed through different locations, such as Compostela, Pontevedra, Madrid, A Pobra, Cambados or Rome, in addition to stays in Latin American countries such as Cuba or Mexico. Among all of them, Madrid played a central role in the writer's life, having a love–hate relationship with it. There he was able to give free rein to his vocation as a talk show host in the many literary cafés of the late 19th and early 20th centuries. He was able to rub shoulders with the intelligentsia of the time, with Rubén Darío, Azorín, Miguel de Unamuno, Pío Baroja or Jacinto Benavente, among others; as well as with prominent politicians such as Manuel Azaña or Natalio Rivas. However, Valle always maintained a dichotomous personality, always divided between the rural and the urban, between modernity and tradition, so his will was to return to his native Galicia.

At the dawn of the spread of the pandemic, Valle-Inclán was in Madrid teaching the chair of Aesthetics at the School of Painting, Engraving and Sculpture, which he held for two years (from 1916 to 1918).[3] He was 52 years old at the time he had been married to Josefina Blanco Tejerina since 1907, and the couple already had three children out of the six, they would engender.

It should be remembered that the pandemic spread across Europe from US soldiers fighting in the First World War; and in Spain, as non-belligerent country, the flu was propagated in Spain through day labourers, religious gatherings and celebrations. It is not trivial to point out that the disease "ha sido catalogada como la mayor pandemia del siglo XX por su extensión geográfica y su incidencia demográfica" (Laguna 2021: 13). In March that year, it began to be very present in this part of the Pyrenees, especially in Catalonia, where educational centres were quickly closed, as Pla recalled. This influenza was highly virulent, affecting all age groups and causing very high mortality, all of which were aggravated by the effects of the last year of the devastating First World War. Once again, literature gives us examples of the ferocity of that flu, since Miguel Delibes in Mi idolatrado hijo Sisí (1953) reflected how it had a devastating impact on the characters and on society "la ciudad entera se sentía atenazada por el invisible fantasma de la gripe. Se dictaron

---

[3] This chair was created ex professo for Valle-Inclán by the government, specifically by the Minister of Public Instruction Julio Burell, acquaintance to the writer. In this way, "el mismo día y en la misma publicación oficial, en sincronía perfecta, que venía a ratificar que el puesto estaba concedido y creado de antemano para don Ramón, el ministro comunicaba al director general de Bellas Artes que el rey había tenido a bien nombrar profesor numerario de la asignatura de Estética a don Ramón del ValleInclán" (Alberca 2015).

una serie de medidas preventivas: secerraron las escuelas y los teatros; se suprimieron los paseos dominicales; las empresas funerarias montaron un servicio nocturno permanente para atender el exceso de enterramientos" (2007[1953]: 551).

Nevertheless, the first wave of the flu (approximately from April to June 1918) was certainly taken lightly in the Spanish capital; as González recalled, "sin embargo, ante la extensión de la epidemia y el cariz que tomaban los acontecimientos el 1 de junio el ABC advertía que era preciso que 'sin alarma, pero con seriedad, dejándose de motes ridículos, que más dicen de inconsciencia que de ingenio, el vecindario se preocupe de la amenaza que le acecha'" (2020).

However, the higher incidence of the virus from May and especially June caused panic to grow in the Madrid where Valle-Inclán lived, although as Alberca reminds us, educational centres were not closed back then, "pero sin duda la vida académica, como cualquier otra actividad, resultó perjudicada. En la Escuela de Pintura, Grabado y Escultura, el ritmo de la actividad docente quedó alterado por el avance de la epidemia: los exámenes se adelantaron, el curso terminó antes y en la escuela hubo desbanda general" (2015). Valle-Inclán and his family participated in this disbandment, since there is evidence that in June 1918 they were already settled in the Merced Pazo, a manor house rented to Xavier Puig in A Pobra do Caramiñal.[4] Thus, in June 1918 Inclán had already left Madrid and had settled with his family in Madrid "ante el peligro de contagio (no se olvide que el matrimonio tiene dos niños), la familia ha optado por salir anticipadamente de Madrid" (Alberca 2015).

In this way, Valle-Inclán spent the summer of 1918 in la Merced pazo from A Pobra, where we remember that he lived intermittently for five years and where he tried to fulfil his dream of living off the land, thus combining his passion for agriculture and literature.[5] In September that year, Valle- Inclán should have already returned to Madrid to rejoin the Aesthetics classes, but by then he was still in the manor house, since the Diario de Galicia echoed a "lively pilgrimage" that was celebrated in it and in which "a portion of distinguished families gave great animation to

---

[4] According to the newspapers of the time, which collected in their pages that Valle was in A Pobra (Diario de Galicia 1918).
[5] Despite this illusion and some income from the sale of vegetables, the cultivation of the vines and the sale of the wine was catastrophic and meant huge economic losses for the Valle family.

the party, being splendidly presented by the gentlemen of Valle-Inclán" ("De la Puebla del Caramiñal" 1918).[6] It turns out how surprisingly was that, in the midst of the second wave of that pandemic, a party was held in the Valle-Inclán's pazo; also, taking into account that from the autumn of that 1918 there would be a second wave much more virulent than the first one.

Continuing with the chronology of that 1918, let us remember that in September that year Valle did not want to return to his position as professor in the chair of Aesthetics in Madrid for different reasons: the flu epidemic, his desire to go to Mexico to investigate and writing a book about Hernán Cortés, as well as for his growing weariness with the teaching task. That is why he insistently requested a leave of absence to visit Mexico from Natalio Rivas, undersecretary of the Ministry of Public Instruction, who suggested that he request a licence. Valle processed it hastily, but in November of that year "cuando finalmente, por orden gubernativa, el curso no se inicie a causa de la gripe, escribirá de nuevo a Rivas para pedirle que deje sin efecto la solicitud de excedencia" (Alberca 2015).[7] Precisely, in communications with Natalio Rivas we discovered that Valle-Inclán contracted the flu in October 1918, during the second wave, a fact that conditioned his confinement on the pazo for about eight months. We reproduce below the moment in which Valle tells Natalio Rivas that he has contracted the flu, the only written document where it can be verified:

> Señor don Natalio Rivas / 13 de octubre de 1918 Mi querido amigo:
> Aunque tardé porque estoy convaleciente de esta maldecida epidemia, me entero de la salida de Alba y entrada del conde de Romanones en Instrucción. No sé si ello traerá dificultades para la realización de mis deseos. A los buenos oficios de usted me encomiendo pues no tengo ninguna suerte de amistad con el nuevo Ministro. Si no pudiesen arreglarse las cosas como usted tenía pensado, apelaré a una excedencia y con ese arreglo me contentaré.

---

[6] In addition, the newspaper's correspondent noted in the note that the vintage that year had been "una mitad que la del año anterior" ("De la Puebla del Caramiñal" 1918), thus testifying to the manifest business failure.

[7] However, the School of Fine Arts demanded that Valle-Inclán join the centre as early as January 1919, reason why he insisted to Natalio Rivas that he need to take leave of absence to travel to Mexico for not starting the course, a fact that translates into a renewal of the licence for, we suppose, illness (letter to N. Rivas 01/2/1919 and 01/24/1919 in Valle-Inclán (2015)).

En suma, fuese ello lo que fuese le agradecería que se solucionase sin necesidad de ir yo a Madrid pues me he quedado un poco delicado y necesito convalecer aquí, y darme un buen calafateo en el monte.

Mi caro y buen amigo perdone toda esta lata. Con el mayor afecto le estrecha la mano. Valle-Inclán. (Carta a N. Rivas 13/10/1918 en Valle-Inclán 2015)

The writer spent two weeks convalescing from the flu in the manor house, maintaining strict confinement in it, as he did not go out to attend funerals or tributes, except on specific occasions.[8] One of the reasons that we can put forward responds to a certain fear of having contracted the disease; the other, without a doubt the main one and our hypothesis, is none other than the inspiration he enjoyed in the solace of the house to write tirelessly. Certainly, the motivation that Valle found in La Merced, in front of the Arousa estuary, explains this prolonged voluntary confinement, since at official level there were no restrictions in this regard. Therefore, we can confirm that Valle-Inclán's confinement due to the flu had a paradoxically productive effect on his literary career, because a year later, in June 1919, he travelled to Madrid to manage the publication of up to five works: Divinas palabras, Farsa de la enamorada del rey, Farsa y licencia de la reina castiza, Cara de Plata, in addition to the best known of his works Luces de bohemia. Thus, Alberca agrees in reviewing that those works are "fruto de este fructífero aislamiento en la Merced" (2015).

Having said that, it is worth asking ourselves to what extent the confinement affected Valle's literary production. On the one hand, the space influenced the prolificacy of Valle-Inclán, that country house in front of the sea surrounded by vineyards, thus "en los años de residencia en La Merced escribió mucho. Fue una de las etapas más productiva, creativa e innovadora de su carrera de escritor [...] En La Merced está escribiendo mucho y eficazmente" (Alberca 2015). Thus, we can suggest that the writer took advantage of this confinement and prolonged it to the maximum due to the happiness and inspiration he experienced in the manor, since "en el pazo de La Merced, don Ramón era más fantasmal que en ningún otro sitio" (Gómez de la Serna 2007: 147).[9] In fact, it is curious

---

[8] Everything indicates that Valle had a mild illness, since there is no evidence of major complications. Let us remember that the author had a somewhat weak health, since he suffered throughout his life from different ailments and operations.

[9] In fact, Valle had always shown his desire to constantly return to Galicia, since, as Gómez de la Serna reminds us "de cuando en cuando se va a sus pazos rotos, desventrados, con la tapia mellada. Era otro Valle en aquellos paisajes saudosos y medrosos.

to remember that in an interview with the writer Vicente Salaverri and published in 1918, Valle-Inclán stated that "yo trabajo espoleado por la fiebre, con facilidad" (1918: 44), statement that helps to reinforce the exposed thesis.

On the other hand, we can glean a deeper influence on the content of Valle's subsequent publications due to the pandemic crisis. The vital pessimism of the moment due to the deaths caused by the flu and the social paralysis of the time permeated the plots and characters of his works. To all this, we must add the impact that the visit to the French front in April 1916 (Alberca 2015) during the Great War had had on him, since the idealization or aestheticism with which he perceived the war conflict quickly vanished when verifying in situ the devastation of the trenches; thus, he "vuelve a España triste. Había visto que la guerra ya no era una epopeya sino algo monótono y feo" (Gómez de la Serna 2007: 134).

As an example, Luces de bohemia stands out for its markedly critical vision of Spanish society sifted through the technique of the esperpento, the grotesque. Let us recall a brief dialogue between the gravediggers of Max Estrella in which this acid vision is perceived: "OTRO SEPULTURERO: En España el mérito no se premia. Se premia el robar y el ser sinvergüenza. En España se premia todo lo malo. / UN SEPULTURERO: ¡No hay que poner las cosas tan negras!" (Valle-Inclán 1924: 262). This deformed and sarcastic depiction of society is connected to and is the corollary of a change in Valle's conception of art. As of 1919, he abandons aestheticism, art for art's sake, and allows himself to be carried away by a socially and politically committed art. In this sense, Cipriano Rivas Cherif, a contemporary writer of Valle, emphasized this change in the Galician author regarding Tolstoy's question ""Qué es el arte": así, D. Ramón no quiere hacer arte puro; pretende hacer historia solamente [...] Inicia con éste [con Luces de Bohemia] una serie de estudios dramáticos, que pudiéramos decir de los fenómenos sociales precursores de la futura revolución española" (Rivas 1920: 4).

In accordance with the foregoing, we agree with Paz in affirming that "el tono pesimista de Luces de bohemia y su visión de la España de entonces posiblemente no sean ajenos al estado anímico en que dejó al

---

Se convertía en trasgo y estafermo y se daba la buena vida que podía, entre boticarios y curas que le admiraban. Se iba a Galicia porque le llevaba allí la morriña y el deseo de ver los pinos sobre el mar y la lluvia sobre la hierba. Era un enterramiento provisional porque no podía más" (2007: 145).

escritor de Vilanova de Arousa aquel virus epidémico tan letal" (2020). This would be, therefore, another of the consequences of confinement and the flu pandemic. However, in the content of his work it is very difficult to glean references to this disease as authors such as Josep Pla or Miguel Delibes did. In our opinion, only the following dialogue in Luces de Bohemia between the Marqués de Bradomin and Max Estrella's gravediggers could be insinuating the high mortality "esta temporada" due to the 1918 flu, which was characterized by also affecting in children, as a gravedigger says:

> OTRO SEPULTURERO: ¡Ya habrá usted visto entierros!
> EL MARQUÉS: Si no sois muy antiguos en el oficio, probablemente más que vosotros. ¿Y se muere mucha gente esta temporada?
> UN SEPULTURERO: No falta faena. Niños y viejos.
> OTRO SEPULTURERO: La caída de la hoja siempre trae lo suyo. (Valle-Inclán 1920: 274)

The hypothesis of this "absence" could respond to a desire to turn the page or to avoid the obvious, the omnipresent, that is, not to delve into a topic that was so traumatic and so vogue at the time. In addition, to end this evaluation of the absence of direct references to the epidemic in Valle-Inclán's work, it should be noted that this was the norm at the time. Science and health were relegated to other types of non-literary texts, since until the 20th century serious illnesses were frequent and writers used to catch ailments such as tuberculosis. Thus, Sampedro and Sánchez affirm that the writers of the turn of the century and the beginning of the 20th century "había influido el romanticismo decimonónico, que trataba la enfermedad de manera simbólica, como una metáfora del enfermar del alma, carente de interés per se. En este sentido, La montaña mágica de Thomas Mann, escrita en 1912 pero no publicada hasta 1924, era el ejemplo más fehaciente de lo anteriormente expuesto" (2020: 479). In this sense, the change towards new narratives related to the disease would take place from the literary renovation promoted by Virginia Woolf or James Joyce and the establishment of a "literature of the disease".

That said, the few references to the flu of 18 that we find in other works prior to Woolf or Joyce are given by different justifications. For example, Pla's work was conceived in 1918 but rewritten and reworked until its publication in 1966. Although, logically, there are specific exceptions that reflect the pandemic in a literary way, such as the case of Eugeni d'Ors, who was also infected with the flu, like so many intellectuals of the time (such as Jaume Brossa) and found himself on the verge of death. Thus, between 8 October and 15 November, he stopped publishing some glosses in La Veu de Catalunya dedicated to great personalities due to the flu (Playá 2020: 37). In addition, he was one of the first writers to make reference at the time through the Glosari relating the flu to the First World War "Ah! Caure sota la metralla vora els plecs de la desplegada bandera! I no en la penombra asfixiant d'una alcova, entre dos llençols suats" (cited by Mas 2005: 82).

Josep Pla and the 1918 influenza pandemic

As we mentioned at the beginning of this study, Josep Pla took refuge from the flu pandemic at his birthplace in Palafrugell. He resided there from 8 March 1918, until returning to the capital of Barcelona on 9 January 1919, according to the dates in The Gray Notebook.[10] The fact is that we cannot say that he was confined in the strict sense as we currently understand it or as Valle-Inclán did. In his case, it was a return to his roots, to the reunion of a calm life to connect with nature and people, for which The Gray Notebook is predisposed as praise to his Arcadia. As we read in the work, it is surprising that Pla did not keep confined in the family home at the height of the pandemic but rather he takes frequent walks, to the hermitage of Sant Sebastià, for example, frequents the coffee bar with his friends, visits relatives or goes on vacation to the beach of Calella de Palafrugell in August 1918, in addition to going to funerals caused by the flu: "al atardecer, voy al café del Centro Fraternal. Encuentro a casi todos mis amigos" (Pla 2016[1966]: 917). This change of life from the big city to the small town is symbolized very well by Pla in reference to alcohol: on 9 June 1918, he refers "en Palafrugell, el alcohol me hace cambiar de vida. En Barcelona me levanto pronto para ir a la Universidad y seguir el curso académico. Llegar aquí y levantarme a las doce en punto es indefectible" (Pla 2016: 2009). Alcohol is nothing less than the contrast between two types of modus vivendi, the sociability and Mediterranean hedonism of Palafrugell versus the dedication and individualism of the big city. Thus, the tone of this work combines gravity due to the ravages of the pandemic while comic touches emerge

---

[10] Specifically, Josep Pla returned to Barcelona on 9 January 1919, after having left due to the epidemic on 18 March. That day he recorded that he went to the University and to the library of the Lawyer's Association.

to exacerbate the physical, hence offering an ironic message about morality: on 14 March 1918, he writes "ahora, finalmente, da gusto vivir en Cataluña. La unanimidad es completa. Todo el mundo está de acuerdo. Todos hemos tenido, tenemos o tendremos, indefectiblemente, la gripe" (Pla 2016: 834).

In the first place, it should be remembered that The Gray Notebook is full of references to the 1918 influenza pandemic, being noteworthy its testimonial and historical value, as well as its literary. It is not trivial that the work begins with a reference to the closure of the University of Barcelona due to the pandemic, since this will be central in the work by conditioning Josep Pla's steps to chance, as we will clarify later. In this sense, Pla begins the diary by referring to 8 March as the day the university was closed due to the pandemic, just to make it anachronistically coincide with the day of his 21st birthday. Later, on 14 March, he jokes about the fact that everyone will be infected; on 9 July he refers to the number of deaths that occur on those dates "cada día pasa por delante nuestra algún entierro" (2016: 2577); on 4 September he hinted at his concern about contracting the disease "cada día me tomo la temperatura" (2016: 3854); on 18 and 22 October, he conveyed his concern about the magnitude of that second wave of the pandemic "la gripe hace terribles estragos. La familia se ha tenido que dividir para ir a los entierros" (2016: 4923) and "la gripe continúa matando implacablemente a la gente [...] Aunque solo fuese por esta razón, convendría que este escándalo de la patología tuviese un fin –que la gripe no matase a nadie más" (2016: 4987).

It is curious, then, Pla's dichotomous testimony in relation to the pandemic in light of two opposite types of life: one hedonistic, without restrictions, and the other focused on constant concern about the disease that suppurates in the lines of The Notebook. In this last sense, on 6 December 1918, the author expresses his terrifying fear of getting infected "por la tarde trato de llegar al mas. Por el camino me siento muy constipado, incómodo, y me pasan unos escalofríos por la espalda gélida. Reculo. Tengo un momento de miedo. Debe de ser la gripe -creo-; si lo es, la muerte es ineluctable" (2016: 5811); Finally, on 24 February 1919, he became infected and alluded to the strong effects that the flu had on him "he pasado todo el día de ayer y una parte del de hoy en la cama, con la gripe. He sudado como un caballo. Treinta y seis horas seguidas. Me levanto pálido y deshecho. Por un lado, me parece que me hubiera podido morir y que me he librado por los pelos" (2016: 7065).

Second, as inferred by the references to the pandemic, two decisive consequences emerge in the literary future of Pla, which we will elaborate here: that pseudo-confinement forged the intellectual foundations of the author at the time when the Empordà landscape became nuclear in his life and work. On one hand, it should be noted that the 10-month confinement in Palafrugell represented Pla's origins as a writer based on the number of works that he was able to read during those months without teaching activity in Barcelona. As we saw before, Pla stated that life in Barcelona implied, at least until January 1919, the sacrifice of attending law classes with which he did not agree. Instead, life in Palafrugell means that he can read works of all kinds without restrictions, from classics to works of the 19th-century French, Castilian or Catalan authors.

In fact, these intertextual references are of great value and give a good account of the enormous number of works that pass through his hands in a relatively short period of time. Pla becomes a voracious reader, and already on 14 March 1918 we find the first sign of intertextuality: "el río pasa y todo me lleva a quedarme, sentado en la ribera. La lectura de las novelas de Baroja -que he devorado, abundantemente, estos últimos días- me ha arrasado los pocos gérmenes de acción que tenía" (2016: 834). It is not surprising that the first literary reference is that of Baroja, for whom Pla will always profess devotion, despite being criticised because he did not develop a memorialist side.[11] In this intertextual network, an author stands out at the other intellectual extreme for Pla: Miguel de Unamuno, whom he describes as a "gibberish".[12] Although the references to Castilian authors are scarce, those related to Catalan and European authors, especially French, are more verbose, an aspect that may respond to the influence of personalities from the literary Ateneu of Barcelona, as the one exercised in Pla Alexandre Plana. In the field of Catalan literature,

---

[11] In another later entry, on 14 October 1918, Baroja is once again emphasised as an essential author in his literary formation "nuestra generación -la generación catalana- debe de haber leído copiosamente la obra de Pío Baroja. A los diecisiete años, yo lo devoraba, y se puede decir que la conozco toda" (2016: 4874).

[12] From Unamuno there is reference to the following reading on 5 January 1919, en su curiosa y divertida Vida de Don Quijote y Sancho -que acabo de leer- Unamuno presenta a Cervantes como un pícaro" (2016: 6238). Moreover, another author in Spanish that Pla stands out is José Ortega y Gasset who affirms on 3 February 1919 that "escribe como un ángel" (2016: 6587). There is also a reference to Azorín, whom he would also meet in Madrid "he leído también un artículo de Azorín sobre Gracián" (2016: 8665) and to Pérez de Ayala on 7 November 1918 "releo Tinieblas en las cumbres, de Ramón Pérez de Ayala" (2016: 5264).

at the beginning of the diary, Pla rushes to quote one of his favourite authors (on 14 March 1918 he reveals that he is reading the Glossary) whom he meets in Barcelona: Eugeni d'Ors or Xènius.[13] Other Catalan authors that he mentions in his diary are his admired Noucentista poet Josep Carner,[14] Jacint Verdaguer,[15] Santiago Rusiñol,[16] Francesc Ferriol,[17] Francesc Pujols,[18] Robert,[19] and even Pompeu Fabra.[20]

To these allusions to authors and reviews of his works, we must add a preponderant mention of European authors, especially French, as well as classics. For example, Pla takes advantage of the period of confinement to read Montaigne incessantly: on 24 April 1918, he comments that "no me canso de leer los ensayos de Montaigne. Así paso horas y horas de la noche en la cama. Me producen un efecto plácido, sedante; me dan un reposo delicioso" (Pla 2016: 1459); then he quotes on 11 October

---

[13] The essayistic aspect of Eugeni d'Ors is what fascinates Pla; on 22 November we find another reference to his reading "en La Veu de Catalunya, Xènius escribe ahora los artículos de La Vall de Josafat" (2016: 5643), as well as on 27 April 1919 "me había hecho el propósito de no leer ningún diario hasta pasados los exámenes. El propósito ha durado muy pocos días. Hoy lo he roto. He leído el Glosari" (2016: 8665).

[14] On 19 March he states that "he leído Les planetes del verdum, de Josep Carner" (2016: 998).

[15] On 24 March he mentions that "de madrugada trato, una vez más, de leer a Verdaguer. No he podido, hasta ahora, terminar ni un solo canto de L'Atlàndida o Canigó" (2016: 1131).

[16] On 26 April he comments that "hace días intento concretar en pocas líneas la impresión que me ha causado una reciente lectura de El poble gris, de Santiago Rusiñol" (2016: 1459); and also on 23 May "en la peluquería leo los escritos que publica en l'Esquella Santiago Rusiñol" (2016: 1858).

[17] On 10 August he asserts that "por la mañana, en el pinar de Ferriol, leo el Dietari de Francesc Ferriol" (2016: 3033).

[18] On 29 October we find "leo el Concepte general… de Francesc Pujols" (2016: 5069), which is described later on 16 December as "es un gran libro, pero es demasiado patriotero" (2016: 5943).

[19] On 1 September 1919 he recounts that "estos días he leído el volumen que la Biblioteca Popular l'Avenç publicó -es el número 73- con algunos artículos de Robert, titulado Barcelonines" (2016: 10854).

[20] On 5 November 1918 he comments that "por la noche leo la Gramática catalana de Pompeu Fabra" (2016: 5215).

M. Joseph Joubert, É. Zola,[21] V. Hugo,[22] Stendhal,[23] G. Flaubert,[24] and H. de Balzac.[25]

Likewise, he mentions other European authors, among which Nietzsche stands out,[26] very much in vogue at that time in intellectual circles; n addition, we find references to J. Jörgensen,[27] L. Tolstoy,[28] G. Leopardi,[29] G. d'Annunzio,[30] F. Dostoevsky,[31] or J. W. Goethe.[32] Finally, we find references to classical authors such as Dante[33] or Plato.[34]

All these references are a good example of Pla's erudition, since he presents himself as a voracious reader in his formative stage, unlike Valle-Inclán. In this sense, the question arises as to where the writer could obtain all these readings during that period of confinement; the answer could be found in his own library filled with works from Barcelona, as well as from the town bookstore, where he left onerous debts, as Pla

---

[21] On 7 November he affirms that "paso la tarde leyendo. Zola está considerado como una naturalista, pero ahora veo, en el Mercure de París, que, al escribir sus novelas, utilizaba muy pocos documentos humanos concretos" (2016: 5264).

[22] On 4 May 1919.

[23] On 8 September 1919.

[24] On 24 February 1919 he expresses that "me causaría un gran placer poder tener las obras completas de Flaubert. Los doce volúmenes de Flaubert valen treinta y ocho pesetas y céntimos" (2016: 7081).

[25] On 8 March, he gives his opinion about this author "Balzac, escritor aburridísimo, pesado" (2016: 7266).

[26] On 15 November 1918 he affirms that "Nietzsche, al que leo en las ediciones publicadas por el Mercure, no me cansa nunca" (Pla 2016: 5661); el 14 de febrero de 1919 "por la noche, en casa, leo Aurora, de Nietzsche" (Pla 2016: 6917); and on 25 February of the same year "me quedo en casa todo el día. Plana tiene la gentileza de enviarme la Vida de Nietzsche de Daniel Halévy" (2016: 7081).

[27] On 15 June he comments that "he leído estos días, el San Francisco del danés Jörgensen" (2016: 2258).

[28] On 9 July 1918 Pla quotes Tolstoi's Diary.

[29] On 20 September 1918

[30] On 15 November 1918.

[31] On 13 December 1918.

[32] On 5 November 1918 Pla states that "la cosa más acertada que he leído sobre política se encuentra en las Conversaciones de Goethe y Eckermann" (2016: 5462)

[33] Quoted on 19 May 1918.

[34] On 19 June 1918 he mentions that "leídas las ochenta y cinco frases que en la traducción francesa de Platón dirigida por Victor Cousin" (2016: 2290); and on 4 November "por la noche, en la cama, vuelvo a los Diálogos de Platón" (2016: 5184).

himself (2016: 5710) attests.[35] Therefore, Plafrugell and the tedious hours of confinement forged his love for reading and promoted the foundations of the future great writer that Pla would become. That is why we find metaliterary comments by Pla in which he bears witness to his will to write and they all converge in the same place: Palafrugell. In fact, the author himself states it:

> Fue la amistad que tuve con Joan B. Coromina, Tomàs Gallart, Joan Linares, Josep Vergés, Josep Ferrer, Josep Miquel, el pianista Roldós, Lluís Medir, Josep Bofill de Carreras, Enric Frigola, Ramon Casabó, y otros que ahora no recuerdo, la que me incitó a escribir. Todas estas personas […] crearon una especie de exaltación palafrugellense, de un localismo vívido y entonces de una curiosidad internacional extraordinaria. (Pla 2016: 11345)

In this way, the confinement due to the 1918 pandemic in his town was decisive in Pla's literary formation and style. For this reason, Soler recalls that the fact of delimiting the geographical space at the beginning of the work is not trivial, but that "l'espectacle que atreia Josep Pla començava i es fonamentava en la seva primera mirada envers aquells contorns empordanesos" (2007: 681). The artialisation of the geography of his native "country", understood as his immediate reality, becomes his artistic predilection through the essay genre. Topography and human geography will become his worldview, a nuclear element in his memorial production, of that atavistic Mediterraneanism that will always appear in his works. This aspect can be seen in the fact that in The Gray Notebook the same landscape is described and narrated on more than one occasion as a result of Pla's walks, emphasising its sensory value for the reader; thus, Comelles affirms that "Pla, doncs, dóna prioritat absoluta a la contemplació, a la descripció, i ens reforça la sensació d'exercici literari que ell mateix explicita" (2016: 324).

Therefore, Pla becomes a homo viator through his region, the Empordà, and his work is configured as a dithyrambic of this region. This is how he expressed in the Diario de Madrid his preference for the description of reality "a mí, por descontado, me gusta la materia, más que nada, la realidad. Siento que la vida del pueblo me acerca a la realidad, a la corporeidad. Descubro en las cosas tal como son el máximo encanto,

---

[35] On 8 November 1918, he confesses his pecuniary problems due to his two passions in Palafrugell: social gatherings and reading: "debo dinero a T. G.; diversos piscolabis; una larga factura al club y una considerable cantidad de libros al librero Lavinya" (Pla 2016: 5710).

elementos de maravilla insospechados" (2020: 199).[36] If we delve deeper into Pla's writings, we come to verify that an article in the Baix Empordà on 3 November 1927 related the origin of his literary vocation to the flu epidemic (Puig 2020: 22). In this sense, his own words reinforce the hypothesis of the relationship between the landscape and the walks, derived from confinement, and his passion for writing:

> Em veig a setze o disset anys, a l'època que hi hagué tanta grip i la Universitat hagué de tancar[37]. Vaig passar tota la tardor i part de l'hivern a Palafrugell. Havent dinat sortia a passejar. Solia pujar a Sant Sebastià. Va ésser en el curs d'aquestes passejades que em sortí a fora la miserable vocació que tinc d'escriptor. […]
>
> No era pas que veiés nimfes darrera dels arbres. De nimfa, no n'he vista mai cap. Era que descobria el món exterior. Tots portàvem, llavors, al costat, sense necessitat d'ésser massa sensibles, la presència de la mort. La malaltia feia estralls, es morien els amics més cars, les cases eren plenes de malalts.
>
> Potser tots estàvem una mica enfebrats. Fou probablement la lucidesa que provoca a estones la por de morir que em féu veure la meravella que tenia al davant. Feia un temps clar, hi havia una llum ideal. Trobava a la terra punts de repòs, recolzades de calma, corbes d'abundància que em produïen una inefable i plena sensació de salut i de seguretat. (Pla 1968: 474)

As Pla himself affirms, that puerile inclination for writing was inevitably marked by the landscape of Palafrugell, especially the path to the Sant Sebastià lighthouse, as well as by the omnipresent fear of death during those months.

In this sense, for Pla the confinement in Palafrugell means to connect with the physical and human geography and make these his worldview. Nevertheless, at the same time, the author perceives the exhaustion of these spaces and needs to expand his gaze to the city and other realities. Seen this way, The Gray Notebook is a kind of bildungsroman in which Pla enters adulthood, which is found in Barcelona, at the university, at the literary Ateneu, in new friendships; and from here to Madrid, to Paris… Pla himself expresses on 26 September the exhaustion – albeit temporary – of the narratives of his people: "encontrándome solo, siento

---

[36] Pla already foresaw that novel would not be the genre he would employ in his future works; hence, in a hunting day he writes that "en momentos así, busco a menudo un argumento de novela. Imposible de encontrar nada. No he tenido nunca bastante imaginación para conseguir ver la vida en forma de novela" (Pla 2016: 5762).

[37] Actually, in The Gray Notebook he states that he is 21.

que en Palafrugell no tengo nada que hacer. Una cierta sorpresa" (Pla 2016: 11082).[38]

Conclusion

As in all historical processes experienced by humanity, literature echoed the serious effects that the 1918 flu had on society. In first place, we have highlighted the value of literature not only from its artistic side but also testimonial and scientific as it is permeable to everyday life. In the second place, we have analysed how this pandemic affected two contemporary authors whose lives and works were conditioned by it. On one hand, both authors were infected with this flu without major consequences for their health, but it was the confinement that made their literary careers develop. We have verified that the confinement was a creative stimulus: in the case of Valle-Inclán the writing of up to five works in just eight months, and for Pla his formative stage with the reading of innumerable classic and contemporary works and the beginning of the outlines of subsequent publications, such as The Gray notebook.

On the other hand, the influence of the landscape was another decisive element that connects both authors, since it contributed to promoting their artistic careers. In the case of Valle-Inclán, his Pazo de la Merced in front of the Arousa estuary and surrounded by vineyards was a balm against the serious epidemic of the moment; Valle left Madrid and strictly confined himself to the manor house, while Pla left Barcelona to seclude himself in Palafrugell but without giving up his social life or the endless walks around the region. In Pla, moreover, those ten months of confinement were the origin and explanation of his work, of his predilection for the essay, for the literary description of physical and human geography.

Finally, we allude to a link between both writers that makes the relationship between disease and literature more tangible. Curiously, both agreed to find the loophole through which to forge their literary careers in the fever and fear of the pandemic. Valle affirmed, not without a touch of sarcasm, "yo trabajo espoleado por la fiebre, con facilidad" (1918: 44); while Pla "potser tots estàvem una mica enfebrats. Fou probablement la lucidesa que provoca a estones la por de morir que em féu veure

---

[38] On 25 September 1919, he passed the subjects needed to complete his law degree.

lameravella que tenia al davant" (1968: 474). In both, the fever, as a literary stimulus, was a warning before death so as to not let the beauty of the world escape.

Bibliography

Alberca, Manuel (2015), La espada y la palabra. Vida de Valle-Inclán, Barcelona, Tusquets, 2015.

Comelles, Salvador (2016), "El caminant i el paisatge. La construcció de les seqüències paisatgístiques en El quadern gris de Josep Pla", Zeitschrift für Katalanistik, 29, 2016, 317–339.

"De la Puebla del Caramiñal" (1918), Diario de Galicia, 27/01/1918.

Delibes, Miguel (1953), Mi idolatrado hijo Sisí, en Obras Completas, Barcelona, Destino, 2007.

Fresnadillo Martínez, María José (2015), "Enfermedades infecciosas en la literatura. Una larga historia sin final", Revista de Medicina y Cine, vol. 11 (1), 2015, 41–53.

Gómez de la Serna, Ramón (2007), Don Ramón María del Valle-Inclán, Madrid, Espasa Calpe, 2007.

González Núñez, José (2020), "La verdadera historia de la Gripe del 18", HoyesArte.com

Laguna Platero, Antonio (2021), Los imaginarios de la gran pandemia de 1918, València, Tirant Humanidades, 2021.

Mas i Solench, Josep M. (2005), Frederic Clascar i Sanou. Entre l'ortodòxia i la política. Barcelona, Publicacions de l'Abadia de Montserrat, 2005.

Paz Gago, José María (2020), "Luces de bohemia frente a la censura", Diario ABC 25/10/2020.

Pla, Josep (1966), El cuaderno gris, en Notas y dietarios, traducción del catalán de Dionisio Ridruejo y Gloria de Ros, Barcelona, Destino, 2016.

–(1957), Dietarios de Madrid, Barcelona, Planeta, 2020.

–(1968), "El genius loci en la meva situació personal i en la meva obra literària", en El meu país, OCVII, Barcelona, Destino, 1968, 474–478.

Playà Maset, Josep (2020), "El tedi, segons Eugeni d'Ors", La Vanguardia, 20/03/2020, 37.

Puig, Evarist (2020), "La grip del 1918 i Josep Pla", Revista de Girona, 321, 22–26.

Rivas Cherif, Cipriano (1920), "Hombres, letras, arte, ideas", La Internacional, 3/09/1920, 4.

Salaverri, Vicente (1918), Los hombres de España, desde Maura al Vivillo, Montevideo, Maximino García, 1918.

Sampedro, María y Sánchez, Guillermo (2020), "La gripe española de 1918 a través de la obra de Laura Spinney El jinete pálido", Revista de medicina y cine, 16, Extra 1, 2020, 469–484.

Slavoj Zizek (2020), Pandemic! Covid-19 Shakes the World, London/New York, Or Books, 2020.

Soler, Glòria (2007), "El paisatge i les afinitats literàries: l'Empordà com a camp de treball literari a El Quadern gris", Annals de l'Institut d'Estudis Empordanesos, 2007, 681–691.

Valle-Inclán, Joaquín (2015), Ramón del Vallé-Inclán. Genial, antiguo y moderno, Barcelona, Espasa, 2015.

Valle-Inclán, Ramón María (1924), Luces de bohemia, Madrid, Renacimiento, Imp. Cervantina, 1924.

"Tourism Yes, Tourism No": The impact of the Covid-19 pandemic on discourse about tourism in the Spanish press[1][2]

DAGMAR VANDEBOSCH – KU Leuven

The role tourism has played in Spanish economy since the 1960s is difficult to underestimate. Since the Franco regime opened up the costa's to foreign tourism, the share of tourism in Spain's GDP increased from about 2 % in 1950 to 12.4 % in 2019 (Vallejo Pousada 2002: 209; INE 2020: 1). Behind this economic growth was a model of massification of tourism and a focus on beach tourism (*turismo de sol y playa*), which in the years leading to the Covid crisis was being increasingly criticised by both academics and local activists, mainly residents and environmentalists. The Covid pandemic had a profoundly disruptive impact on Spanish Tourism, pushing back the sector's share in the GDP to 5.5 % in 2020 and causing an acute economic and social crisis in the sector, which revealed the risks of the country's strong dependence on tourism.

This chapter aims to analyse the impact of the Covid crisis on discourse about tourism in mainstream Spanish press in the two years following the crisis of March 2020, more concretely from the start of the pandemic in March 2020 to mid-April 2022, i.e. the beginning of the *Semana Santa* or Easter period, traditionally the first seasonal peak in Spanish tourism. The analysis takes into account both the editorial discourse of the newspapers and the opinion pieces published in their columns and focuses on three topics: the reporting of the economic and social consequences of the pandemic in the tourism industry, the reflection on the future of tourism in Spain, and the fate of the controversy about the touristic model and its social and environmental impact in a (post-)pandemic context.

Four Spanish newspapers have been selected for this study: *ABC*, *El Mundo*, *El País* and *La Vanguardia*. This selection represents the four

---

[1] This chapter was realized thanks to the funding of FWO-Flanders.
[2] "Turismo sí, turismo no", *La Vanguardia* 22.06.2020.

most-read daily papers in Spain and covers a broad sample of Spanish society, both geographically and ideologically (Enguix Oliver 2023: 153). While *El País*, *El Mundo* and *ABC* are national, Madrid-based papers, ABC also has a historically strong presence in Seville. *La Vanguardia* is a Catalan newspaper, published in Barcelona in Spanish.[3] In Spain's highly politicized media landscape (Casero-Ripollés 2012: 31–32), these papers also span moderate left-wing (*El País*) and more conservative views (*ABC, El Mundo*). The case of *La Vanguardia* is somewhat particular in this regard, in the sense that its editorial line was generally considered conservative, but its association with Catalan nationalism strongly opposes it to *El Mundo* and *ABC*, the latter being overtly monarchist in addition. In the period which concerns us, and in the years immediately prior to the pandemic, the question of independence came to be the main fault line in Catalan politics, transcending traditional political boundaries and gathering left- and right-wing parties in a pro-independence coalition government.

In what follows, I will first sketch the controversy about tourism in Spanish social discourse previous to the pandemic, before studying the way in which the impact of the corona crisis is presented in the corpus.

Before the crisis: Criticism and *"turismofobia"*

In the first decade of this century, the social and environmental impact of massified tourism became a topic of scholarly study, on the one hand, and of citizen activism, on the other hand. As Novy and Colomb show, these contentions about tourism occurred in cities worldwide and tended to involve the same economical, physical, social, cultural and psychological sources of conflict (2017: 19–20). In Spain, critical attitudes towards the existing model of touristic exploitation and the discourse of touristic growth were particularly strong in Barcelona and the Balearic Islands, two of the main touristic destinations, which in the course of the first two decades of the 21st century also saw a shift towards a so-called "low-cost tourism", with the rise of low-cost airlines and online renting platforms such as Airbnb or HomeAway. Particularly between 2015 and 2020, the harmful impact of "overtourism" or touristic saturation (Milano 2017: 6)

---

[3] Since 2011, *La Vanguardia* also has an edition in Catalan. For this research only the Spanish edition has been used.

became an important topic in academic publications and in social discourse. Geographers, sociologists, anthropologists and ecologists increasingly focused on topics such as the impact of tourism on the housing market (gentrification, expulsion of locals from the city centre) and on the environment. In the broader society, associations of local residents regularly organised manifestations to protest against the pressure tourism put on their neighbourhood (Milano 2017: 30–32, Mansilla López y Hughes 2021, Novy and Colomb 2017: 3). Several non-academic books published in this period address the unwanted or damaging effects of tourism, such as *Viaje al turismo basura* (2016) by journalist Joan Lluis Ferrer, the more pamphletary collection *Jodidos turistas* (2017), and, to a certain extent, Marina Garcés's *Ciudad princesa* (2018).

The genre that arguably has been most effective in raising awareness on the topic, nevertheless, has been the documentary. Eduardo Chibás's film *Bye Bye Barcelona* (2014) was the first to address the issue, with a montage of interviews with academic experts and citizen representatives and of footage that visualizes the massification of tourism and the vulgar commodification of culture (Gaudí, flamenco, etc.). This film focuses mainly on the so-called *parquetematización* of the city, that is, the transformation of public space into an attraction park for tourists, instead of a living environment for residents. The interviews address the social impact of "touristic rental" (*alquiler turístico*), by which apartments are rented to touristson daily basis, taking them out of the housing market for local residents and often causing problems of cohabitation between tourists and permanent occupants, especially since Barcelona became a cherished destination for "booze tourism" (*turismo de borrachera*). Other issues addressed are the restraints on the use of public space, either by privatization (Park Güell) or by congestion (Ramblas, neighbourhood of Sagrada Familia). Over the last five years, several other documentaries have criticised the existing model of tourism for its destructive impact. In 2018, Laura Álvarez directed *City for Sale*, which documents the impact of tourism on the lives of four local residents who face expulsion from their houses. *Tot inclòs* (2019) and *Overbooking* (2019) tackle the impact of tourism on the Balearic Islands. In addition to the impact on the housing market and the urban space, these films focus on the environmental costs of the tourist industry on the islands through the pressure on construction, water and energy consumption, waste management and transportation (particularly rental cars and cruise ships). Another "new" topic they address is the precarity of the employment in the sector, with a particular interest in the working conditions of the cleaning staff of hotels. This interest can be directly linked to the movement of the "Kelly's" – short for *"las que limpian"* ("those who clean"), an association of chambermaids whose struggle against outsourcing, exploitation and, more recently, in favour of a more ethical form of tourism had received quite some public attention and gave rise to another documentary, *Hotel Explotación: las Kellys* (2018). The last documentary made before the pandemic, *Destrucció creativa d'una ciutat* (2020), addresses tourism in a more indirect way but equally focuses on the disruptive impact of gentrification in the popular neighbourhoods of Palma de Mallorca.

It is interesting to observe that the more "participatory" of these documentaries (Nichols 2010: 180) are places in which academic discourse stands aside activist and citizen discourse, since both parties are being interviewed on their expertise and experience. Academic and activist discourses are even more intertwined in the case of *Tot Inclòs. Danys i conseqüències del turisme a les nostres Illes*, an annual journal edited by the collective *Tot inclòs*, which is also behind the documentary of the same name. This journal, which presents itself as an ecologist and anticapitalist activist publication, contains contributions of both social and environmental activists and academics, such as geographers Albert Arias Sans and Ernesto Cañada. Geographer Ivan Murray published articles in *Tot Inclòs* using the pseudonym of Eliseu Casamajor but does claim these articles as his on Research Gate.

In the summer of 2017, tourism became the object of a polemic in Spanish media, which evolved around the concept of *"turismofobia"*. The immediate cause of the polemic was a series of acts of vandalism and provocation against tourism infrastructure committed by Arran, a political group of Catalan independentist, socialist and feminist youth. Reactions condemning these acts labelled them as sings of *"turismofobia"*, a term which had been circulating for about a decade among defensors of tourism but was not frequently used until the 2017 polemic.[4] In their analysis of 40 contributions to this polemic, mainly opinion pieces and interviews published in a wide range of media, Raquel Huete and Alejandro Mantecón (2018: 15–16) distinguish two highly polarized and antagonistic discourses, which they label as "legitimizing" and "critical"

---

[4] Huete and Mantecón (2018:12) trace the origin back to a 2008 essay by José Antonio Donaire, while Milano (2017: 28) attributes the term to Manuel Delgado in an article published in *El País* in the same year.

discourses on tourism. Two elements in this analysis deserve pointing out: (1) the political, rather than professional affiliation and motivation of these contributions, which in the case of the "legitimising" pieces are of the hand of representatives of the governing right-wing Partido Popular and to a lesser extent of entrepreneurs in the touristic sector, while the critical opinions are attributed to Arran and Ernai, the youth sections of left-wing independentist movements in Catalonia and the Basque Country and, in their less combative variants, to associations of residents; (2) the entanglement of arguments relating to tourism with political or ideological issues, such as independentism or class struggle. This seems to corroborate Novy & Colomb's views on tourism as a topic that is easily politicized and the contestation of which "revolve less around tourism itself than around broader processes, policies and forces of urban change" (2017: 4). It is unclear to which extent Huete and Mantecón's conclusion about the absence of a "discursive structure" situated in between the two antagonistic discourses (20121: 16) applies to the discourse on tourism after the polemic of the summer of 2017, which ended abruptly, as the authors recall, with the terrorist attacks on the Ramblas on 17 August. According to Mansilla López and Hugues (2021: 40–41), the fear of the anti-tourism campaigns of 2017 generated a shift in political discourse on tourism towards a focus on hospitality and tolerance (*discurso de la convicencia*), on the one hand, and sustainability, on the other hand – a shift which, as I shall explain below, also is related to changes in the Spanish government and in European policies. A quick view on the publications in *El País* over this period shows that the discourse defending the benefits of the tourist industry, which was dominant until about 2017, makes way for more critical articles which take into account social and environmental impact of tourism.[5]

While certain scholars (e.g. Zerva et al.) use "*turismofobia*" in a non-problematic or descriptive way to refer to critical stances towards tourism, I agree with Huete and Mantecón that the concept is too politicized and connoted to have any analytical value. I will also refrain from using terms

---

[5] e.g. Ruiz Plantilla, Jesús, "Marina Garcés: "El turismo es la industria legal más depredadora" (entrevista), *El País* 13.08.2018; Vázquez, C., "Los vecinos de Valencia se plantan con las terrazas y los

pisos turísticos", *El País* 23.01.2019; Blanchar, Clara, "Los vecinos somos una especie en peligro de extinción", *El País*, 27.07.2019; Toharia, Mar, "Hacia nuevos modelos de turismo urbano", *El País* 10.09.2019; Molina, Margot, "El frágil equilibrio entre turismo y conservación", *El País* 28.02.2020.

such as "antitourism" or "anti-touristification", which reflect an activist position that is not uncommon in Spanish academia (e.g. Mansilla and Hugues describe their perspective as that of a researcher-activist (*perspectiva investigadora-activista*) (2021: 33)). Instead, I will speak of "criticism" or "critical perspectives" on tourism, in order to include in the research many critical reflections that question aspects and modalities of the touristic industry, rather than reject tourism as a whole. In this sense I agree with Novy and Columb that rather than "a global 'revolt against tourism' […] we are seeing a proliferation of forms of contestation – big and small – surrounding tourism. However, given their oftentimes different causes, characteristics and concerns – and taking into account that many of them are not *against* tourism as such – one should avoid the pitfall of making them appear more similar or uniform than they are in reality" (2017: 4–5).

Social and economic impact of the Covid crisis

Turning to our journalistic corpus then, the first striking observation is that a majority of articles about tourism in all four newspapers in the two years following the outbreak of the Covid-19 pandemic focus on the economic impact of the crisis and its social consequences. This is of course no surprise, since the touristic sector was particularly affected by the lockdowns and restrictions on mobility, which reduced international travel almost entirely and domestic travel considerably in 2020 and whose impact was still felt in 2021. All newspapers follow up on statistics-monitoring processes of decline and recuperation of touristic activities, made public by the National Institute of Statistics or by the sector itself.[6] These quantitative data are often accompanied by updates on the financial aids offered by support measures of the national government or by EU funding. The Spanish government resorted to a system of temporary unemployment, known as ERTE (Expedientes de Regulación Temporal

---

[6] Some examples of such articles: Aguilar Madrid, Jorge, "El turismo perderá casi 100.000 millones

de euros este año", *ABC* 19.05.2020; Villaécija, Raquel, "El turismo 'adelgaza' del 12,4 % al 4,3 % en el PIB", *El Mundo*, 21.01.2021; Suñé, Ramon, "El turismo retrocede a niveles de hace 20 años en Barcelona", *La Vanguardia*, 07.010.2022; Galindo, Cristina, "España recibe un 64 % más de turistas en 2021, pero sigue lejos del nivel previo a la pandemia", *El País* 02.02.2022.

de Empleo) in order to assure "flexibility and stability of jobs",[7] while the European Union also set out to boost tourism in its post-pandemic recovery plan NextgenerationEU,[8] albeit with the conditions of making tourism more green and digital. Especially in *El Mundo* and *ABC* the government, a coalition of moderate and more radical left-wing parties, is criticised for doing too little too late[9] and for maintaining discouraging security measures in the summer of 2020, while other European countries did open up to international tourism.[10] *La Vanguardia* publishes two more extensive, in-depth articles on the impact of the crisis on employment. "¿Adonde fueron todos aquellos empleos?" puts the current crisis in an disillusioning historical perspective, comparing the current Covid-driven shift of jobs in the tourist sector towards more precarious and unstable contracts in food distribution or domestic service, with the shift of the stable on relatively well-paid jobs in the Catalan textile manufactories of the 1960s and 1970s towards less attractive positions in tourism, after the outsourcing of textile production to Asia.[11] The second article, a long report based on interviews, focuses on the movement of the chambermaids or "Kelly's" (cf. supra), presenting them as "victims of the pandemic".[12] It recapitulates the claims and struggle of the women prior to the crises and sketches the harsh circumstances in which the abrupt closing of the hotels has left them, drawing particular attention to the fate of the many workers who, lacking a fixed position, were not eligible for temporary unemployment payments (*ERTE*). *La Vanguardia*'s interest in this collective contrasts with the lack of interest in other media and

---

[7] https://www.sepe.es/HomeSepe/erte-red .
[8] https://europa.eu/next-generation-eu/index_en .
[9] Aguilar Madrid, Jorge, "La falta de ayudas al turismo amenaza el liderazgo de España tras la crisis", *ABC* 04.05.2020; Villaécija, Raquel, ""El Gobierno llega tarde. Hay que reconstruir el turismo" (interview with Jorge Marichal), *El Mundo* 14.10.2020.
[10] Iriarte, Marcos, "Alerta turística: Grecia destrona a España como destino con más reservas de cara al verano", *El Mundo* 19.02.2021; Ginés, Guillermo, "El turismo español constata una fuga de viajeros hacia países más abiertos'", *ABC*, 12.07.2020. The headline accompanying this article is even harsher, stating that "El turismo agoniza en España mientras la UE abre sus fronteras", accompanied by a photomontage showing the leaders of Germany, France, Austria and Italy holding an "Open" sign, while Spanish prime minister Sánchez's board reads "Closed".
[11] Aymerich, Ramon, "¿Adónde fueron todos aquellos empleos?", *La Vanguardia* 14.03.2021.
[12] Sampedro, Sergio, "La otra cara del turismo de Benidorm: el largo invierno de las 'kellys'", *La Vanguardia* 01.02.2021.

the facetious and arguably misogynous tone used in *El Mundo* to report on the decision of the Balearic president Francina Armengol to force hotels to improve working conditions for their cleaning staff:

> Entre otra serie de medidas, [Armengol] prometió obligar a la industria hotelera a adaptar sus hoteles para favorecer al colectivo de empleadas de la limpieza, instalando camas elevables. La medida se presentó ante la mirada y el aplauso de la ministra de Trabajo y vicepresidenta segunda del Gobierno, Yolanda Díaz, afín a Armengol y pública defensora del movimiento de las kellis [sic], como se autodenominan las camareras de piso.[13]

El Mundo dedicates articles to the devastating economic impact of the crisis on the sector in general[14] and in several subsectors of tourism, such as the hotel and catering industry,[15] travel agencies[16] or rental cars.[17] In its coverage of the social consequences of the crisis, it resorts to human interests stories with rather bold headlines, which mention twice the "hunger queues" (*colas de hambre*)[18] in which the people most affected by the crisis stand in line for free food. A similar focus on the economic impact and human interest approach of the social consequences of the crisis can be found in *ABC*. *El País*, as we shall see in the following section, tends to focus more on recovery and change in the sector.

ABC does stand out in its coverage of the impact of the crisis on housing and real estate. While *El País* and *El Mundo* treat the *hausse* of hotels that are being put for sale in a rather neutral and descriptive way, *ABC* adopts the perspective of the financial sector, elucidating the motivation of companies trying to sell real estate in order to remain solvent and of

---

[13] Colom, Eduardo, "Baleares pone el turismo en pausa", *El Mundo* 12.02.2022.

[14] Iriarte, Marcos, "Los salarios sufren su mayor caída en medio siglo y arrasan el turismo", *El Mundo* 02.03.2021, as well as a large number of interviews with business people, particularly CEOs of hotel chains, and representatives of the public sector.

[15] Rocés, Paco C. "Adopta un bar: paga copas y cenas por adelantado para que no cierre", *El Mundo* 02.05.2020.

[16] Hernández, María, "El SOS de las agencias de viajes", El Mundo 05.12.2020; García, Isabel, "El renacer de las agencias de viaje a causa de la pandemia", *El Mundo* 22.05.2021; Villaécija, Raquel, "El lento resurgir de las agencias: tres de cada 10 trabajadores siguen en ERTE", *El Mundo* 13.02.2022.

[17] Villaécija, Raquel, "El Covid deja sin coches de alquiler a los turistas de Baleares y Canarias", *El Mundo* 06.08.2021.

[18] Espinosa, Javier, "Canarias, del 'boom' turístico a las colas del hambre", *El Mundo*, 18.01.202; Colom, Eduardo, "Colas del hambre en Baleares: del maná del turismo a pedir para comer", *El Mundo*, 01.02.2021.

financial funds attempting to buy hotels at dumping prices. One contribution presents the crisis as an opportunity for financial investment. In the same line, the decrease of housing prices in the coastal areas is perceived as a menace to the refuge value of the construction sector.[19] *La Vanguardia* offers a completely opposite view on a rather similar issue, that is, the increasing attempts of international investment funds to purchase vacant commercial properties in the centre of Barcelona, treating them as opportunists who take advantage of the turbulent times.[20] This phenomenon is presented as an undesired effect of a strong delay in the recovery of the commercial city centre, which, according to the journalist, can be ascribed not only to the pandemic but also to the restrictions the city government imposes on commercial activities in the centre of the city, and to the pressure of low-cost tourism, which leads to further degradation of the commercial supply in the city centre. As a Catalan regional paper, *La Vanguardia* shows a double preoccupation for the disruptive economic impact on a region which is far more dependent on tourism than the country's average, on the one hand, and the potentially harmful impact of a return to mass tourism on urban life and on the environment on the other. Both preoccupations give rise to quite extensive articles about the future nature of tourism and about the flaws of the current model. I will comment upon these texts in the next sections.

For now, I would like to focus on one particular aspect of the social impact of the crisis: the fall of renting prices. This subject receives attention in *El País*, *El Mundo* and *La Vanguardia*. It is attributed to two causes: the shift from touristic to conventional residential renting as a result of the decrease in tourism due to the pandemic, and, in the case of Barcelona, the impact of legal restrictions on touristic rental since 2020. While lower renting prices and a larger residential offer are considered positively in a context of socio-economic hardship, journalists remain

---

[19] Colmenero, Ricardo F., "Más hoteles en venta que abiertos", *El Mundo* 23.10.2020; Cía, Blanca, "Los hoteles en venta en Barcelona se disparan con la pandemia", El País 07.12.2020; Aguilar Madrid, Jorge, "El número de hoteles en venta en España se dispara de un 30 % en un año", *ABC* 10.08.2021; Aguilar Madrid, Jorge, "Es un momento ideal para invertir en hoteles", *ABC* 20.10.2021.

[20] "Son los oportunistas, que son un montón, pescando en río revuelto". Benvenuty, Luis, "El turismo 'low cost' demora la reactivación comercial del centro", *La Vanguardia* 03.07.2021; "Los pisos de la costa se deprecian sin turismo", ABC 21.08.2020.

sceptic as to the duration of this effect.[21] More interestingly perhaps, the question of legal regulations of renting prices meets with surprisingly little resistance in *El Mundo* and *ABC*, papers which tend to privilege economic interests over claims of city residents affected by tourism. An editorial piece in *El Mundo* deems regulation "necessary for tourists flats", not only because they contribute to rise of renting prices and the expulsion of residents from the city centre but also because they engage in unfair competition with the hotel industry and lead to urbanistic degradation.[22] Pieces in *El Mundo* and *ABC* on a bill launched by the socialist President of the Autonomous Community of the Balearic Islands, which plans a moratorium on tourist flats, criticise the fact that the bill was passed by decree in order to avoid a parliamentary vote but do not openly disagree with its content (although *El Mundo* treats it rather sarcastically). Finally, *La Vanguardia* celebrates these regulations and reports on the first conviction for illegal subletting to tourists in Barcelona as a victory over an "illegal tourist accommodation mafia".[23]

The impact of the pandemic on tourism in Spain was of such weight that it comes as no surprise that almost no attention is given to the situation in other, especially non-European, countries with a well-developed tourist industry. The only exception is *El País*, with contributions on the impact of the Covid crisis in tourism in African and Latin-American countries, and an extensive article on resilient, sustainable and equitable tourism in Mexico.[24]

---

[21] "La caída del turismo provocada por la pandemia ha hecho que se pusieran más viviendas en el mercado convencional, pero este hecho puede ser coyuntural" (Suñé,Ramon, "Aumenta el número de alquileres y bajan los precios en Catalunya", *La Vanguardia* 06.03.2022). José Luis Aranda reaches a similar conclusión in *El País* ("Los pisos turísticos elevan hasta un 19 % la oferta de alquiler residencial", *El País* 07.06.2020 and "El alquiler turístico se prepara para el fin de la pandemia", *El País* 18.07.2021).

[22] "[…] los pisos turísticos, que actúan tantas veces como agentes de competencia no regulada de empresas hoteleras y que están teniendo un impacto considerable en las ciudades españolas, sobre todo en las zonas céntricas. Son un factor que ha contribuido a la expulsión de vecinos estables hacia otras áreas, y a que se disparen los precios del alquiler habitacional" ("Regulación necesaria para los pisos turísticos", *El Mundo* 14.08.2020).

[23] Benvenuty, Luis, "Condena ejemplar por realquilar pisos a turistas", *La Vanguardia*, 04.04.2022.

[24] Nadal, Paco, "Sin turismo hay hambre", *El País* 11.06.2020; Nadal, Paco, "¿Cómo sería el mundo sin turistas?", *El País* 18.02.2021; Meneses, Nacho, "Sostenible, equitativo y enriquecedor para todos: así será el turismo del futuro", *El País* 03.12.2021.

The future of tourism

The sudden shutdown of tourism in the spring of 2020 drew attention to one problem related to tourism that eclipsed the issues discussed in the years before, and that was the country's extreme, and in some regions almost exclusive, economic dependence on the sector. All newspapers critically examine the economic flaws of the existing "quantitative" touristic model, whose main objective consisted in maximizing the number of visitors, and which ended up monopolizing the economy in the principal touristic regions. This last phenomenon, which in critical academic and social discourses on tourism had often been described with the agrarian metaphor of "monoculture" (*monocultivo*), is referred to in economics as "the Dutch disease". The Corporate Finance Institute defines Dutch disease as "a concept that describes an economic phenomenon where the rapid development of one sector of the economy (particularly natural resources) precipitates a decline in other sectors".[25] This concept is used in a contribution by Pedro Aznar, professor in economics, in *La Vanguardia* that summarises the insights of all four newspapers as an effect of the pandemic:

> muchas zonas turísticas se enfrentan a lo que se conoce en economía como la enfermedad holandesa. Cuando un sector productivo aumenta de modo considerable su peso en la actividad económica, acaba desplazando otras actividades, como la industria, de forma que ese territorio no tiene los activos, infraestructuras, ni la oferta laboral, en términos de formación de sus empleados, que favorezca la inversión en otros sectores. Vislumbrar alternativas al turismo no es imposible, pero si enormemente difícil en el corto plazo.[26]

This difficulty of finding viable economic alternatives to tourism on a short term probably explains why pleas for a decrease in tourism are rare in our corpus. One exception needs to be mentioned: in the early summer of 2020, Juan Antonio Pavón Losada publishes an opinion article in *El País* stating that "a decrease in tourism already was necessary before [the pandemic], but is an absolute priority

---

[25] https://corporatefinanceinstitute.com/resources/knowledge/economics/dutch-disease/#:~:text=Dutch%20disease%20is%20a%20concept,appreciation%20of%20the%20domestic%20currency.

[26] Aznar, Pedro, "El futuro del turismo se enfrenta a la 'enfermedad holandesa'", *La Vanguardia* 29.04.2021.

now".[27] The author denies that tourism generates wealth and urges his country not to relapse into the old habits of uncontrolled building, corruption and social, cultural and environmental degradation. Instead, efforts should be made to reorient the economy towards more beneficial and resilient activities in the areas of industrialisation, digitalization, innovation and new technologies.

However, journalists, opinion makers and interviewees, from Barcelona's mayor Ada Colau in *La Vanguardia* to Antonio Garamendi, President of the Spanish Confederation of Enterpreneurial Organisations, in *El País*, agree on the necessity of a quick recovery of the sector and a fundamental turn to different and more sustainable forms of tourism.[28] The reflection on the future of tourism in the four papers of our corpus gives rise to a reflection on the tourism of the future. Sustainability, digitalization, diversification and deseasonalization are key concepts in this process and are actively stimulated by the national government, and in the case of the first two concepts, by the NextGenerationEU recovery fund (cf. supra).[29]

Diversification and deseasonalization often go hand in hand and were already presented before the crisis as a means of diminishing the dependence on massified beach tourism and shrinking the gap between high and low season. After the crisis, all the papers in our corpus explore new or "different" forms of tourism under the motto "Quality before quantity": cultural tourism,[30] responsible tourism,[31] rural tourism,[32] sports

---

[27] "El decrecimiento turístico ya era necesario antes, pero ahora es una prioridad absoluta". In Pavón Losada, Juan Antonio, "La vuelta del turismo post Covid-19: una oportunidad de cambio", *El País* 12.06.2020.

[28] "Hay que recuperar el turismo, y que sea sostenible" (interview with Ada Colau, *La Vanguardia*, 30.05.2021; Garamendi Lacanda, Antonio, "Por una recuperación del turismo con visión de futuro", *El País* 17.09.2021.

[29] The most extensive and elucidating article on NextGenerationEU, which also pays attention to steps already taken by private sector, is Óscar Granados's article "¿Cuáles son las claves para revitalizar el turismo?", *El País*, 12.07.2021.

[30] Llanos Domínguez, María, "Turismo cultural: la puerta a la España de las oportunidades", *ABC* 12.04.2022; LV 30.05.2021.

[31] Fluxá Thienemann, Sabina and Gloria Fluxá Thienemann, "Turismo responsable: la clave para reconstruir una industria mejor", *El Mundo* 05.06.2020.

[32] Nef, Andrés, "El turismo rural de Girona sale reforzado de la crisis turística", *El Mundo* 05.10.2021.

tourism,[33] mountain tourism[34] and regenerative tourism.[35] These forms of tourism are not only more sustainable but also more prone to attract domestic tourism as well as wealthier tourists who are expected to behave in a less disruptive manner. A particular type of "quality tourism" is luxury or "premium" tourism, aimed at the highest segment of the market, often in non-European countries. This is the card played by the PP-led government of Madrid in the last years, which receives quite some attention in the three nationwide newspapers.[36]

While digitalization is frequently cited as a future goal, it seldom gets in-depth coverage. A brief mention was made in ABC regarding a partnership between the World Tourism Organization and the Spanish telecom firm "Telefónica". This collaboration aims to utilize big data analysis and AI to enhance differentiation, personalization, and security in the tourism sector. A more detailed article on this topic can be found in La Vanguardia, which highlights the application of AI, Big Data, augmented and virtual reality, and biometrics in the realm of tourism.[37]

Sustainability, on the other hand, is omnipresent in these reflections on future tourism. Several articles differentiate between economic, social and environmental sustainability – three approaches that tie in perfectly with the EU's plan to orientate the recovery from the pandemic towards a "green", "digital", "healthy", "strong" and "equal" Europe.

Although all four newspapers dedicate ample attention to sustainability, their framing of the subject differs considerably. While *El Mundo*

---

[33] Muñoz Vita, Ana, "El Covid impulsa un turismo deportivo más responsable", *El País* 26.11.2021; Álvarez, Ramón, "La millonaria conexión entre turismo y deporte", *La Vanguardia* 21.10.2021

[34] Qu, Dongyu, "Reconstruir un turismo más sostenible en las montañas para las personas y el planeta", *El País* 11.12.2021.

[35] Ortí, Antonio, "Adiós a la turismofobia: el turismo regenerativo mejora el viaje y el destino", *La Vanguardia* 16.11.2020.

[36] Domingo, Marta R. "La capital, a la caza del turista 'premium' para apuntalar la recuperación", *ABC* 31.08.2021; Peinado, Fernando, "Un camarero del Four Seasons gana mucho más que uno del 100 Montaditos", *El País* 11.08.2021; Gutiérrez, Hugo, "El turismo de lujo resiste a la pandemia", *El País* 07.11.2021; Gómez, Virginia, 'Más hoteles de lujo y un museo del fútbol para sumar turistas", *El Mundo* 12.04.2022. *ABC* dedicates no less than six articles to touristic planes in Madrid; only the most comprehensive is quoted here.

[37] "Alianza entre Telefónica y la OMT para que la inteligencia artificial impulse el turismo", *ABC* 02.06.2021; Valero Carrera, Alicia, "Cuatro tecnologías para salvar al turismo", *La Vanguardia* 04.08.2020.

and *ABC* tend to see the shift towards sustainable forms of tourism as an economic necessity and/or opportunity, *El País* and *La Vanguardia* frame it as an opportunity to find solutions to economic, social and environmental challenges. *El Mundo* often quotes extrinsic motivations for this shift, such as European funds and international tendencies,[38] and tends to approach topics from a classic financial-economic perspective in which sustainability is not a core value. The four objectives that Inmaculada Benito – director of Tourism, Culture and Sports in the Spanish Confederation of Entrepreneurial Organizations – presents in the tribune "Hacia un nuevo turismo", for instance, show little proof of a substantial change in direction. While "generating touristic value in interaction with other economic sectors" might be considered as a sustainable remedy for the "Dutch disease", "consolidating Spain's international position", "making use of European funds" and "public - private collaboration" are classic recipes. Nor does social sustainability have a place in Benito's discourse, which presents only companies and consumers as interested parties, leaving out other social partners (employees, residents, etc.).[39] Even an article about a regenerative agricultural programme on Mallorca frames sustainability in an economic logic, as a way of regenerating the islands by exploring their "natural capital" and focuses primarily on its financial organizational model.[40]

El Mundo's predominantly economic focus is also reflected in the interviews and opinion pieces published on the matter. *El Mundo* dialogues intensively, as do *ABC* and *El País* to a smaller extent, with leading politicians and business people from the sector. *Mutatis mutandis*, these findings correspond with those of Salvador Tejedor et al., who in a comparative study of European newspaper headlines on the Covid-19 pandemic situates Spain, on the basis of an analysis of *El País* and *El Mundo*, among the countries with the largest mediatic presence of public figures, rather than sanitary staff or people affected by the disease (2021: 268–269). In relation to tourism in times of the pandemic, *El Mundo* publishes interviews with the CEOs of AC Hotels by Marriott,

---

[38] "La pandemia ha hecho que muchos países se replanteen su modelo turístico de sol y playa, más masificado. El Parlamento Europeo está otorgando ayudas a proyectos que fomentan el turismo sostenible." In Villaécija, Raquel, "Viejo y nuevo turismo para disfrutar Europa", *El Mundo*, 01.06.2020.

[39] Benito, Inmaculada, "Hacia un nuevo turismo", *El Mundo* 07.08.2021.

[40] Fresneda, Carlos, "Cómo regenerar las Baleares: del monocultivo del turismo que se desmorona a diversificar y reverdecer las islas", *El Mundo* 28.10.2020.

the Meliá group and RIU hotels; with Inmacudala Benito, the director of Tourism, Culture and sports of the Spanish Confederation of Entrepreneurial Organizations; and with Alberto Garzón, the minister of Consumption, whose unfavourable comments on the tourism sector in May 2021 caused great controversy (cf. infra). If we compare this to *El País*, we also see interviews with executives of the hotel sector, and a tribune of Antonio Garamendi, the president of the Spanish Confederation of Entrepreneurial Organizations. *El País*, however, publishes more contributions of academics, political communication specialists (such as the already mentioned Juan Antonio Pavón Losada) and representatives of intergovernmental organizations. These contributions not only focus on sustainability as an economic factor but also as a social, ecological and even a political matter. Indeed, some articles in *El País*, and also one contribution in *ABC*, signal the need of political unity of "bringing together a very atomized sector" and coordinating policies on a local, regional, national and European level.[41] These contributions mostly offer a moderate and balanced view on the shift towards new forms of tourism and take into account different aspects of sustainability. The definition three geographers of the University of La Laguna on the Canary Islands offer of sustainability as "the whole of harmonizing criteria of economic growth, employment and well-being" is a good illustration of that position.[42] Another example is Qu Dongyu and Zurab Pololikashvili's piece on mountain tourism, which mobilises economic, environmental, social and "ethical" arguments.[43] In *El País*, ecological and social or "equitable" (*equitativo*)[44] sustainability receive attention, even in articles whose primary focus is not environmentalist.[45]

---

[41] Noceda, Miguel Ángel, "Entre la Q de calidad y la Q de sostenibilidad y seguridad", *El País* 23.01.2022; Peralba Fortuny, Raúl and Manuel Butler Halter, "El turismo tras la pandemia: ¿y ahora qué?", *El País* 24.06.2021; Barciela, Alberto, "El turismo que ha de volver", *ABC* 18.01.2021.

[42] "[…] la sostenibilidad —entendida como conjunto de criterios armonizadores del crecimiento económico, el empleo y el bienestar—". In Hernández, Jesús, Serafín Corral Quintana and José Luis Rivero Ceballos, "Turismo, crecimiento y cohesión económica y social", *El País* 02.06.2020.

[43] Qu, Dongyu and Zurab Pololikashvili; "Reconstruir un turismo más sostenible en las montañas para las personas y el planeta", *El País* 11.12.2021.

[44] Meneses, Nacho, "Sostenible, equitativo y enriquecedor para todos", *El País* 03.12.2021.

[45] Muñoz Vita, Ana, "El Covid impulsa un turismo deportivo más responsable", *El País* 26.11.2021.

La Vanguardia, as we have seen in the previous section, stands out for its interest in matters of social sustainability, particularly with regard to employment, as illustrated in the articles on the Kelly's and on the downward evolution of qualitative jobs in Catolonia over the last 50 years.[46]

Criticism and *turismofobia* during and after the crisis

One last question to be addressed is whether the dominant focus on economic downfall and recovery and on the futureproof transformation of tourism has banned the existing critical discourse from the columns of our newspapers and, if this is not the case, whether it is still being framed in polemical terms.

The corpus shows a clear division in regard to this question, between *El País* and *El Mundo*, which steer clear of the "old" debates surrounding tourism, on the one hand, and *ABC* and *La Vanguardia* on the other hand, which do reengage with these arguments, and even occasionally frame their intervention in reference to the "*turismofobia*" polemics.

The periodicals of the first group, *El Mundo* and *El País*, focus on the present-day crisis and the future of tourism without overt references to the debates about social and environmental impact of the model of massified beach and "booze" tourism. They strongly differ, however, in the extent to which they politicize tourism. According to Andreu Casero-Ripollés (2012: 33) the strong politization in Spanish media is not so much due to direct links with political parties but rather to the pressure within media groups who use their media to protect their own business interests and to interact with other, mainly political, elites (Curran, in Casero-Ripollés 2012: 34–35). In an traditionally two-party system, this lead to what Sampedro and Seoane (2008) have labelled "antagonistic bipolarization", in reference to the transferral of the permanent, negative and personalized political campaign onto the media coverage of the elections of 2008. While *El Mundo* does not engage in politicized debates on tourism, its coverage of political decisions regarding the sector, particularly by left-wing authorities, is strongly politicized and negative. One example is the already quoted article about Francina Armengol's bill imposing

---

[46] Aymerich, Ramon, "¿Adónde fueron todos aquellos empleos?", *La Vanguardia* 14.03.2021; Sampedro, Sergio, "La otra cara del turismo de Benidorm: el largo invierno de las 'kellys' ", *La Vanguardia* 01.02.02021.

restrictions on touristic accommodations and establishing standards for ecological sustainability and working conditions for the cleaning staff in the Balearic Islands. This article does not thoroughly discuss the content of the bill but rather discredits it using a suggestive and sarcastic tone, stating that the government "basically freezes the creation of hotel rooms [...] in an eminently touristic region, which received more than 16 million visitors in 2019", and by drawing ample attention to the "close" relation between Armengol and the communist Minister of Work and Social Economy Yolanda Díaz.[47] A second illustration is the interview with Alberto Garzón, the radical left-wing Minister of Consumption, whose derogatory statements in the current tourism industry as being "precarious", "seasonal" and of "little added value" unleashed a media storm in the spring of 2021. This interview leaves ample space for the interviewee to make its point and does not use negative strategies, but its many questions about the Minister's "communist" views, as well as the reference to the decoration of his office, in which pictures of executions of the insurgents against Charles V hang next to the portrait of king Philip VI, do frame it in an antagonistic way.[48] Interestingly, critical postures on tourism in foreign contexts appear in a non-politicized way, or even adopt the perspective of the collectives of citizens *El Mundo* tends to ignore in a national context. Irene Hoez Velasco's article on the tourism in Venice in the era of Covid, for instance, criticises the Italian government for having ignored a problem which is presented as so obvious that UNESCO is considering to rate the threat of tourism to Venice's patrimony as comparable to that of war:

> Se trata de algo que las organizaciones ecologistas y medioambientales, las fundaciones de protección del patrimonio artístico veneciano y, en general, la humanidad entera reclamaban desde hace años, pero que sólo ahora el Gobierno italiano ha aprobado. Y, en gran medida, porque se ha visto contra las cuerdas, porque de no hacerlo existía la fortísima posibilidad de que la Unesco incluyera a Venecia en la lista negra de Patrimonios de la Humanidad

---

[47] "Es decir, se congela la creación de habitaciones de hotel y plazas para el alquiler vacacional hasta el año 2026 en una región eminentemente turística, que en 2019 recibió más de 16 millones de visitantes." In Colom, Eduardo, "Baleares pone el turismo en pausa", *El Mundo* 12.02.2022.

[48] Segovia, Carlos, "Alberto Garzón: 'Habrá que reducir el déficit mediante más ingresos y no vía recorte de gastos'" (interview with Alberto Garzón), *El Mundo* 13.06.2021.

en Peligro, junto a países como Siria, Afganistán o Yemen, asolados por guerras.[49]

In *El País,* the arguments and voices which dominated the debate in 2017 and found some echo in the paper in the years after the polemic move to the background as a consequence of the crisis. A brief analysis of references to the polemic in the scarce articles alluding to the subject, suggests that, in the eyes of *El País*, the debate indeed belongs to the past: "La pandemia lo ha trastocado todo, pero *antes de que apareciera este virus existía una corriente de turismofobia,* una cierta sensación de que el turismo se nos había ido de las manos"[50] [my emphasis]. Another of these articles, Paco Nadal's report on abandoned tourist destinations, collects interviews with experts on tourism and with representatives of the Assembly of Neighbourhoods in favour of a Decrease of Tourism (ABDT) in Barcelona. For neither of them, the empty streets of the city are a motif for optimism. The ABDT bitterly states that the sudden fall of tourism lacks any of the positive consequences a planned transition from "monoculture" to a more diversified and fair economy could entail, while the experts see little evidence of a paradigm shift. Breaking with his role as a mere reporter, Nadal takes side and subscribes to their pessimist views:

> Si quieren mi opinión, difiere poco de la de ellos. Tenemos una oportunidad única para corregir errores. Pero no la vamos a aprovechar. Volveremos a viajar, sí. Pero igual o peor que antes. Los humanos somos así.[51]

More frequently, however, *El País* makes a plea for the intellectual and formative value of travel and tourism. An article by Guillermo Alteres, in which the social and ecological drawbacks and the destructive potential of tourism receive distinct critical attention, intertwines this information with reflections of writers and academics on the benefits of travel.[52] Another eulogy of travel is found in an interview with Mario Vargas

---

[49] Hoez Velasco, Irene, ""La última plaga sobre Venecia", *El Mundo* 06.09.2021.
[50] Nadal, Paco, "El turismo es la mejor defensa contra la caricatura de los otros" (interview with Mario Vargas Llosa], 12.02.2021. The article by Nadal and Alteres quoted in the following notes also suggest polemic abruptly put an end to the debate about the drawbacks of tourism.
[51] Nadal, Paco, "¿Cómo sería el mundo sin turistas?", *El País* 18.02.2021.Ibíd.
[52] Alteres, Guillermo, "Por qué merece la pena seguir viajando", *El País*, 09.07.2021.

Llosa, who, when asked whether tourism is destructive, defends it as a crucial dam against cultural prejudice:

> el turismo es absolutamente fundamental, no solamente por el goce que significa conocer otras culturas, otros paisajes, sino fundamentalmente para vencer los prejuicios, los prejuicios que están tan profundamente arraigados en nosotros respecto al otro.[53]

The same idea is formulated by Tony Wheeler, the founder of Lonely Planet, in an interview with *ABC*.[54] Xenophobia, in fact, is presented in several contributions in *ABC* as a characteristic of so-called "*turismofobia*", a term *ABC* uses without reservations to refer to critical approaches to tourism. In an editorial of April 2021, Minister Garzón's negative comments on tourism are described as the "exhibition of a prejudice of the extreme left against foreign tourism".[55] In the same text, the editors state "the left doesn't seem to care about the xenophobic and rancid image" their criticisms project.[56] An opinion piece by writer Xavier Pericay adds an ingredient to the ideological cocktail, namely nationalism:

> No es de extrañar [...] que en el archipiélago [the Balearic Islands] los dardos izquierdistas hayan tenido siempre como objetivo el sector turístico. Unos dardos, por cierto, en los que no ha faltado el componente xenófobo aportado por los nacionalistas del lugar, deseosos de ver su tierra limpia de forasteros, ya sean estos españoles, ya de otras latitudes.[57]

"Nationalist" is in this text considered as synonymous to "xenophobic"; criticism on the hegemonic touristic model, in its turn, is strictly associated to the radical leftist parties who are part of the coalition supporting the independence of Catalonia. This gives rise to the following equation: "*turismofobia*" = communism = independentism = nationalism = xenophobia.

Discourse on tourism is in *ABC* frequently and strongly politicized in a way that reminds Sampedro and Seoane's antagonistic bipolarization.

---

[53] Nadal, Paco, "El turismo es la mejor defensa contra la caricatura de los otros" (interview with Mario Vargas Llosa], 12.02.2021.
[54] Sánchez, Carlos Manuel. "Entrevistas. Desafíos XL". *ABC*, 24.01.2021.
[55] "[...] la exhibición de un prejuicio propio de la izquierda extrema contra el turismo extranjero", in "Urge recuperar el turismo", *ABC* 03.04.2021.
[56] "A la izquierda parece no importarle la imagen xenófoba y rancia que transmiten sus críticas". Ibíd.
[57] "Pericay, Xavier, "Bendito turismo", *ABC* 12.07.2020.

The already mentioned editorial piece, for instance, accuses left-wing voices criticising the decision of the PP-led government of Madrid to attract French teleworkers in plain Covid crisis, of hypocrisy for not condemning the arrival of German tourists in PSOE-governed Mallorca. Especially in opinion pieces, the tone can be harsh, aggressive and personal: "a nadie le escapa que la parte chavista y comunista del ejecutivo comulga con la doctrina antiturismo. Ada Colau, que es un libro abierto, viene anticipando la ideologización de las políticas públicas".[58] Strikingly, most of these articles do not deny the problems addressed by the critics, but they either try to "put them in perspective"[59] and/or express their conviction these problems will be dealt with in the future by stricter regulations.[60]

La Vanguardia is the newspaper in our corpus in which the critical discourse on tourism most strongly persists during the crisis and the early phases of recovery. Articles dealing with the economic and social impact of the pandemic often echo existing criticism. The preoccupation with the strong dependence on tourism, for instance, evokes the indictment of tourism as a form of "monoculture" (cf. supra), showing how the impact of the crisis on local commerce is enhanced by the impoverishment of the variety of shops in the city centre due to tourism,[61] or arguing that the city needs to invest in culture in order to avoid the centre turning into a "ghetto".[62] In addition, as soon as tourism starts to recover in 2021, the complaints of residents about antisocial behaviour of tourists find their way to the columns of *La Vanguardia*, both in articles by their own journalists[63] and in opinion pieces, such as the one of Maria Rodriguez Castilla, who thinks it is "sad we forgot our resolutions of the

---

[58] Girauta, Juan Carlos, "Cómo destruir una economía", *ABC* 16.05.2020.

[59] "Se puede mejorar mucho del sector?... sin duda. Como en toda la vida. Sobre todo en los aspectos laborales. Y hay que ponerse a ello en cuanto salgamos de esta". In Pérez, María Jesús, "Es el turismo, estúpidos", *ABC* 17.05.2020.

[60] "Es de creer [...] que con el tiempo los organismos públicos terminarán por regular ambas modalidades turísticas [cruise ships and tourist flats], dada la necesidad de fijar, socialmente hablando, unos límites razonables". In "Pericay, Xavier, "Bendito turismo", *ABC* 12.07.2020.

[61] Benvenuty, Luis, "El turismo 'low cost' demora la reactivación comercial del centro", *La Vanguardia* 03.07.2021.

[62] Molina, Miquel, "Para evitar que el turismo arrase con todo", *La Vanguardia* 30.05.2021.

[63] Benvenuty, Luis, "El turismo 'low cost' crispa a los vecinos de Barcelona", *La Vanguardia* 18.08.2021.

pandemic so soon".[64] To a certain extent, this position is countered by Ramon Aymerich, who warns against speaking about tourism in moral terms: being an economic activity, it needs economic solutions.[65] This spread between acknowledgement of the economic importance of the sector and recognition of the residents' claims becomes obvious in an article about the city centre of Valencia. After interviewing two collectives, one defending a small, qualitative and sustainable form of tourism, the other one stating they "don't miss tourism" and campaigning against the privatization of public space, Raquel Andrés Durà is unable to answer the question whether tourism is positive or negative for the city centre.[66]

Does *La Vanguardia* participate in the politicization of discourse on tourism? Contrary to *ABC* or *El Mundo*, it avoids antagonistic, negative or personalized discourse about a perceived political adversary. However, both the profile of interviewees (Ada Colau) and opinion makers and the choice of topics of interest, such as the history of degradation of employment in Catalonia or the movement of the Kelly's, reflect an affinity with the (radical) left.

Conclusions

In this chapter one has studied the impact of the Covid-19 crisis on discourse about tourism in four major Spanish newspapers in the two years following the outbreak of the pandemic (March 2020–April 2022). In the years before the crisis, tourism had been the object of strong criticisms, mainly from academics and residents in cities and regions affected by the negative impact of massified and "low cost" tourism, which had

---

[64] "Es triste que se nos hayan olvidado tan pronto los buenos propósitos de la pandemia. Uno de los importantes fue depender del turismo y menos del turismo barato, es decir, una parte del británico. Si este no viene, habremos de buscar no otros turistas, sino otra forma de turismo". In Rodríguez Castilla, María, "Turismo barato", *La Vanguardia* 21.06.2021.

[65] "Lo que no se puede hacer es hablar del turismo en términos morales. El turismo es una actividad económica y si hay cosas que fallan, hay que trabajar para arreglarlas". Gutiérrez, Maite, "Ramon Aymerich: "Barcelona ya no puede vivir sin turismo" (interview with Ramon Aymerich), *La Vanguardia* 19.05.2021.

[66] "Así que, ¿el turismo es positivo o negativo para el centro de València? Lo que está claro es que la pandemia ha visibilizado que es necesario abrir el debate sobre el modelo para el futuro y sobre la búsqueda del difícil equilibrio entre turismo-vecindario." In Andrés Durà, Raquel, "Las dos caras de la caída del turismo en el centro de València", *La Vanguardia* 23.07.2021.

unchained a polemic between "critics" and "legitimizers" of tourism fought out mainly in the media. In this debate, criticism of the hegemonic touristic model was frequently labelled by its defenders and by the press as a phobia – "*turismofobia*".

Our research has showed that the outbreak of the pandemic indeed shifts the attention of the media towards the immediate economic and social impact of the crisis on the one hand (downfall and, later on, recovery, of the touristic industry; loss of employment and social measures; impact on the housing market), and towards the need of changing the current economic model, making the "tourism of the future" more sustainable, qualitative, diversified and digital, on the other hand. In this way, the Covid crisis, which raised awareness of the risks of extreme economic dependence on the sector, in combination with a left-wing national government sharing some of the critical views on tourism, and the conditions of sustainability and digitalization imposed by the NextGenerationEU funds, contributed to a shift in the dominant model. In some of the newspapers, particularly *El País* and *El Mundo*, this leads to a weakened interest in the debates surrounding local impact of tourism. In *ABC* and *La Vanguardia*, instead, events such as the derogatory comments of Minister Garzón on the value of the tourist industry (*ABC*) or the misbehaviour of drunken tourists in Barcelona (*La Vanguardia*), provoke reactions which mobilise the same arguments used before the crisis. In three of the papers, tourism is politicized to a certain extent, as can be expected of a topic that is "easily politicized" (Novy and Colomb 2017: 4) in a strongly politicized media landscape (Casero-Ripollés 2012: 33). This tendency is strongest and most explicit in *ABC*, with overt comments on political parties and politicians. In *El Mundo* and *La Vanguardia*, political motifs may explain the choice of perspective, topics and interviewees. Lastly, *El País* avoids political framing of the topic.

Bibliography

Casero-Ripollés, Andreu (2012). "El periodismo político en España: Algunas características definitorias", en *Periodismo político en España: concepciones, tensiones y elecciones*, Casero-Ripollés, Andreu (ed.), *CAL: Cuadernos Artesanos de Latina*, 33, 19–46.

Enguix Oliver, Salvador (2013). *Periodismo político en España: de la academia a las portadas de la prensa. La hegemonía política de las primeras páginas de*

'El País', 'El Mundo' y 'La Vanguardia' en contraposición a la enseñanza del periodismo político en las universidades españolas, Doctoral tesis, Universitat de València.

Huete, Raquel & Mantecón, Alejandro (2018), "El auge de la turismofobia ¿hipótesis de investigación o ruido ideológico?, *Pasos*, vol. 16 n.1, pp. 9-19.

INE (Instituto Nacional de Estadística). *Cuenta Satélite del Turismo de España (CSTE). Revisión estadística 2019* (press note). 11.12.2020, 1–4. https://www.ine.es/prensa/cst_2019.pdf.

Mansilla López, José Antonio and Neil Hughes (2021). "'En dos años no nos vamos a acordar de la pandemia'. Análisis del discurso sobre el decrecimiento turístico en Barcelona", in *Barataria. Revista Castellano-Manchega de Estudios Sociales*, 30, 30–52.

Milano, Claudio (2017). *Overtourism y Turismofobia: Tendencias globales y contextos locales*. Barcelona: Ostelea School of Tourism & Hospitality.

Nichols, Bill (2010). *Introduction to Documentary*. Bloomington: Indiana University Press.

Novy, Johannes and Claire Colomb (2017). "Urban Tourism and its Discontents", in *Protest and Resistance in the Tourist City*, Colomb, Claire and Johannes Novy (eds.), London: Routledge, 1–30.

Tejedor, Salvador, Laura Cervi, Fernanda Tusa Jumbo and Marta Portalés (2021). "La información de la pandemia de la Covid-19 en las portadas de los diarios. Estudio comparativo de Italia, Reino Unido, España, Francia, Portugal, Estados Unidos, Rusia y Alemania", in *Revista Mexicana de Ciencias Políticas y Sociales*, 242, 251–291.

Vallejo Pousada, Rafael (2002). "Economía e historia del turismo español del siglo XX", in *Historia Contemporánea*, 25, 203–232.

Zerva, Konstantina, Saida Palou, Dani Blasco and José Antonio Benito Donaire (2019). "Tourism-philia versus tourism-phobia: residents and destination management organization's publicly expressed tourism perceptions in Barcelona", in *Tourism Geographies*, 21 (2), 306–329.

The inhumanity of neoliberalism and of the far-right in the context of the Covid-19 pandemic in Brazil

CÉSAR BOLAÑO *(Federal University of Sergipe)*
FABRÍCIO ZANGHELINI *(Federal Fluminense University)*

Introduction

The failure of the "new modalities of capitalist domination" after the Second World War (Bihr 1999 [1991]: 37), in the 1970s, is evidence of the disintegration of the social pact that governed the period of the so-called "welfare state" and the inauguration of the neoliberal project that dominated the 1980s. Furthermore, since the turn of the 21st century, historical social achievements of the working class have been increasingly under attack by the legacy governments of the so-called new right, which, while paradoxically brandishing a critical discourse of "leftist" policies carried out by moderate neoliberal governments, radicalized the neoliberal directive under the veil of defending nationalist, conservative and anti-systemic agendas.

In the case of Brazil, this trend has been fully exploited even in the face of the pandemic reality of Covid-19. The Bolsonaro government, with the support of a significant part of the business community, the military and neo-Pentecostal churches, is waging an extensive war against social policies, customs and science, exemplified mainly by its behaviour during the current public health crisis. Hence, this chapter seeks to explain the link between the neoliberal project and the ideological extremism of the Brazilian government in the pandemic context by showing how the apparently irrational discourse of denial is actually part of a political strategy in service to the radical neoliberal project implemented in the country.

By addressing a historical perspective, the first section of this chapter seeks to reveal how, beginning with the June 2013 protests or "journeys" (as they have been called), the Right has progressively gained prominence in the streets. It will also address how the conservative movement that constituted the social base of the 2016 institutional coup has been advancing, from the arrest of the former president Lula and the victory of the far-right candidate in the 2018 elections. The second section analyzes government actions and strategies related to the Covid-19 pandemic and seeks to explain the preservation of the neoliberal project of privatizing the country's Unified Health System ("Sistema Único de Saúde" – SUS) throughout the entire process. The third section presents data that explain the dramatic result of those strategies, compared with other countries, in terms of contamination rates and the number of deaths resulting from Covid-19.

The conclusion is that neoliberal radicalization in Brazil, occurring between 2018 and 2022, led not only to the deepening of the economic and social crisis already installed in 2013, which assumed the shape of an institutional crisis already in 2014, resulting in the legal-parliamentary coup of 2016, but also to a major health catastrophe, aggravated by the destructive strategy of the Brazilian state adopted by the neoliberal far right in relation to educational, scientific, technological, cultural, ecological, social, labor and social security policies. The text ends with some considerations about Brazil's position in relation to vaccines and the subservience of the Bolsonaro government to the US government led by Donald Trump.

From the 2013 protests to the 2018 elections: The advancement of neoliberalism and the far-right in Brazil

In June 2013, large acts of social mobilization were held on the streets of many of the biggest cities in Brazil to protest against the increase in public transportation fares. These demonstrations were initially led by the Movimento Passe Livre (MPL), a decentralized social organization lacking any political party apparatus. One of the main causes embraced by the almost decade-long movement was fighting for a Zero Tariff in public transport in several Brazilian cities (Bolaño, Cabral and Vaz, 2014). The acts, which were organized and widely publicised through social networks, quickly aggregated several social sectors and new popular claims, revealing that, according to Demier (2015), "their slogan included claims and demands that went beyond the fragmented syndicalism that that had previously characterized a great part of the struggles in the former period".

Laying emphasis on the role of social networks, Machado and Miskolci (2019: 950) compare the June 2013 demonstrations with the so-called Arab Spring, the Occupy Wall Street movement, and the Spanish *Indignados* movement, which erupted in the early years of the 21st century. The comparison arises from the fact that these demonstrations relied on "the ease of sharing content, the popularity of personal profiles and, above all, the power of algorithms to attract attention, muster support to political causes, and thus induce political action" (Machado and Miskolci 2019: 950). The authors therefore state that, despite the existence of previous movements that had also made use of social networks, such as the Marijuana Marches, SlutWalks and other demonstrations in the country, the June protests stood out for demonstrating the extent in which "the political use of commercial social networks generated impact that reverberated throughout society" (ibid.).

However, without denying the importance of the use of Information and Communications Technology (ICT) to these movements regarding its potential as a tool at the service of organization and propaganda, one must not forget, as cautioned by Bolaño, Cabral and Vaz (2014: 20), that "the fundamental plane is political and economic with respect to the construction and preservation of the conditions of cultural autonomy by the social movement". In this sense, this autonomy must be questioned, not only from the viewpoint of its relationship with state powers but fundamentally, with regard to the association between working-class organizations, on the one hand (positive), and the ability to manipulate those who have the corporate media and other institutions at the service of hegemony, on the other (negative). In retrospect, if one considers, nowadays, both the Arab Spring and the various demonstrations supported the lawfare processes in Latin America at about the same time, or even the so-called color revolutions in Eastern Europe, including that of 2014 in Ukraine, it appears that this autonomy was extremely questionable.

Up until that point, the 2013 protests were not directed exclusively against the Federal Government, as they addressed all political parties and politicians equally, both of whom were discredited in terms of their ability to solve basic problems. Largely due to police repression authorized by mayors and governors across different party lines, demonstrations became "viral on the internet, thus triggering the occurrence of other demonstrations" (Demier 2015). In a few days, as it turned out, the protests spread to a national scale and popular dissatisfaction went beyond the issue of public transport, as the discussions expanded to encompass the lack of investment in public services in general. Moreover, this sentiment was reinforced as the population became aware of the hefty investment granted by federal and state governments in construction projects related to major sporting events: the 2014 Football World Cup and the 2016 Olympic Games (Bolaño, Cabral and Vaz, 2014).

In essence, the "increase in public transport tariffs represented the last straw for workers and the low-income population, giving vent to accumulated indignation" (Bolaño, Cabral and Vaz, 2014: 16), given that the last two Labor Party (PT) administrations, despite the advances when it came to social inclusion, failed to break with the structural pillars of neoliberalism and with the income and wealth concentration that characterizes Brazilian society. The inclusion strategy itself, without changing the consumption pattern that illustrates Brazil's historically excluding development model, broadens the expectation horizon (to borrow Celso Furtado's expression), the fulfillment of which would require structural changes that did not occur. In this sense, it is true that the PT government in 2013 did not know how to listen to the clamor of the streets, but they were not given enough time, as we shall soon see.

As usual, the mainstream media attempted to influence public opinion and steer the course of the protests. At first, reproducing the discourse of city mayors and state governors, the press considered the protests to be uncivilized and tainted by vandalism by "highlighting the inconvenience caused by the protests rather than the demands" of the protesters (Bolaño, Cabral and Vaz, 2014: 18). However, as soon as they understood that there was a potential dispute over the control of the streets, which could weaken the Dilma government, the commercial media swiftly inflected and began calling the demonstrations civic and democratic acts. At the same time, extreme right-wing and ultra-liberal groups, which were being consolidated in Brazil, realized the moment and the conditions were right to try to exert their influence over the social movement, in the sense of promoting a change of regime through acts staged by entities such as *Vem Pra Rua* ("Come to the Streets") and MBL - *Movimento Brasil Livre* ("Free Brazil Movement"), influenced by institutions such as "the *Instituto Liberal* (The Liberal Institute) and *Instituto von Mises* (Von Mises Institute), which began publishing pamphlets and magazines, releasing books translated from classical liberal thinkers, and holding large events" (Finguerut and Souza 2018: 245).

The violence of the middle class articulated in this conservative bloc and the manipulative actions of the hegemonic media managed to change the focus of the demonstrations and their sociological characteristics to such extremes that, at a certain point, the MBL, which was present at the origin of the process, decided to withdraw. The movement ended up acquiring overtly right-wing characteristics and adopted the same hackneyed rhetoric against corruption that characterizes these sectors in all coup-inclined processes throughout Brazil's republican history. Jessé de Souza (2014: 46) reminds us that it was "the middle class who took to the streets in masses [...] and was responsible for changing the agenda [...] in favor of their claims centered on corruption allegations – always personalized and state-derived". In the same sense, Demier (2015) states that the ideology of an eminently corrupt political system is "constitutive of the Brazilian *democratic-shielded* regime. Its function in this is, above all, to remove the subaltern segments of the so-called 'political system', leaving it entirely free and available for capital managers".

President Dilma, at first, understood the nature of and reasons for the demonstrations and signaled the correct path by defending an Exclusive Constituent. However, faced with the hesitation of her own party and the opposition of the ruling classes, she maintained the policy of governability and even promised to adopt the measures defended by conservative liberalism, namely: political reform, anti-corruption acts and fiscal responsibility. As a result, in addition to missing the opportunity to get closer to the social movements, which were initially of a popular nature and, for that reason, involved forces that could have fostered structural reforms, the government ended up proposing measures that benefited the right-wing sectors in the following years, such as the creation of the National Public Security Force and the passing of the Anti-Terrorism Bill, thus stifling further potential for a more radical change.

Despite these troubles, President Dilma Rousseff managed to be reelected in 2014, albeit by a narrow margin. This led the set of actors, including the previously mentioned right-wing institutions and movements and the mainstream corporate media, as well as the most significant part of the political class and important sectors of the legal system, to adopt a decidedly coup-inclined strategy. Regarding the demonstrations that took place during the first months of 2015, now led by the far right, they somewhat reproduced the *Marches of the Family with God for*

Liberty, which mobilized the civilian base of the 1964 military coup. In 2014, a movement called *Operação Lava Jato* ("Operation Car Wash") started being articulated in the Brazilian judiciary, and the media coverage powerfully collaborated in shaping public opinion in favor of the impeachment of the elected president.

If no crime of fiscal responsibility had been committed to justify an impeachment, one had to be invented and that's precisely what happened.[1] This complex process will not be analysed here, but today there is broad consensus that what followed was a legal-parliamentary coup; in other words, an institutional rupture in Brazilian liberal democracy, with a coating of legality, since it proceeded in accordance with the rites of due process of the Federal Congress and under the seal of the Federal Supreme Court (STF). In this scenario, Vice-President Michel Temer assumed the presidency with the explicit aim of applying radical neoliberal policies, which basically translated into waging a demolishing war on labor rights (Bolaño and Zanghelini 2022) and freezing the primary expenditures of the public sector (health, education and all claims of 2013 movements), leaving the state free to allocate resources for the benefit of public debt and in service of financial capital.

Furthermore, according to Soares (2018: 24–25), there was a regressive attempt at public health reform in the Temer administration, as well as "authorization for the privatization of aquifers, progress in the privatization process of Petrobras […] development of a draconian social security project", facilitating the sale of property to foreign capital. Furthermore, there was a military intervention, under the legal argument of "ensuring law and order", in the city of Rio de Janeiro. During the intervention period, however, there was no progress in terms of public safety in the city; on the contrary – the period culminated in the assassination of councilwoman Marielle Franco, a murder case that has yet to be solved.

The greatest beneficiary of the new situation was a previously rather obscure politician from Rio de Janeiro, Jair Bolsonaro, who was able to mobilize a broad base of the far-right across the country and make good use of the political climate and, above all, to win the support of national

---

[1] Flimsy charges of "fiscal backpedaling" – a common accounting technique that involves temporarily re-managing funds owed to public banks to cover specific deficits of social programs – characterized the alleged responsibility crime against the Chief Executive Officer.

elites and North American imperialism. He managed this by promising to deliver control of the economic policy to the ultra-liberal economist and banker Paulo Guedes, in addition to nominating the anarcho-capitalist Roberto Campos Neto for the presidency of the Central Bank. It is worth noting that Guedes was part of the economic team of the Chilean dictator Augusto Pinochet, and Campos Neto is the de facto (and political) heir of the most famous economist of the early years of the Brazilian military dictatorship. Thus, the economic policy of Bolsonaro's government represents continuity with Michel Temer's, but is even more radical, as seen from the example of promoting the autonomy of the Central Bank, among other measures.

However, for this transition to proceed according to plan, there was a problem that needed to be solved first: the presidential candidacy of the former president Luís Ignacio Lula da Silva, who was favored in the electoral polls for the 2018 election. The disenfranchisement of his political rights and his arrest as a result of Operation Car Wash constitutes an exemplary case of lawfare, as recognized worldwide, without which the 2016 coup would not have been completed (Uchôa 2022).[2]

Considering the progression of the far right in the Brazilian political landscape, Calil (2020: 82) notes that the period between 2013 and 2018 is not "yet another chapter of the polarization between the PT [Workers' Party] and PSDB [Social Democratic Party] that has marked Brazilian politics since 1994". It is, rather: "the composition of a third pole, founded on anti-establishment rhetoric and which did not hesitate to assume extremist positions such as the defense of 'constitutional military intervention'. Amid this process, in 2017, a clear shift was visible in

---

[2] It is not secondary to point out, as Uchôa (2022: 143) explains, that the United States showed energetic involvement in the institutionally destabilizing events that have occurred since June 2013, mainly in relation to the Operation Car Wash plot. Among other things, there is strong evidence of "deals between *Lava Jato* prosecutors and US Department of Justice prosecutors", which characterizes the coordinated actions of various elements of the so-called hybrid wars. Although President Lula had an apparently amicable relationship with the Obama administration, Uchôa (2022) also highlights, when referring to an interview given by former Foreign Minister Celso Amorim, that this unconventional war was being engendered in opposition to a possible newfound sovereignty produced by pre-salt reservoirs found in Brazil and the closer proximity of Brazil to the other BRICS countries (namely, Russia, India, China, and South Africa).

the configuration of the Brazilian political spectrum, especially evident in social networks widely employed by the far right".

The idea of a third pole emerging refers merely to what occurs when there are disputed options in the electoral game and is debatable, from the point of view of a class analysis, since the far right alternative has historically always been present and held power for long periods of time, mainly during the 1964 to 1985 military regime. The author highlights (Calil 2020: 77) the ideological strategies used to ingrain a worldview that is "individualistic, conservative, moralistic, entrepreneurial, privatizing and meritocratic. Articulately, they advanced concepts based on social and moral conservatism, permeated by sexist, misogynistic and homophobic concepts, relying on expressive resources and a solid organizational structure".

Calil (2020), however, does not discuss the material conditions that would allow for such a radical shift in voters' worldview. The lack of a class-based perspective, in turn, prevents the author from perceiving the fact that it is not a question of constituting a third pole, but a radicalisation movement of voters that had traditionally voted for the PSDB party. Besides, this movement managed to achieve continuity (and depth) both during the 2018 elections and in the current course of events, since Operation Car Wash was unmasked, given the Supreme Court's suspicion of Judge Sergio Moro's partiality, leading to the cancellation of all legal proceedings against the former president Lula, who subsequently returns to the first position in the 2022 electoral polls.[3] The novelty in the current polarization is the existence of a significant portion of voters who

---

[3] For the author, there is "another aspect" that would explain "the intensity with which conservative ideas advanced: lack of resistance from the popular camp, resulting from the frailty of organizations and apparatuses connected to the working classes, which in turn was caused by the institutionalization and transformism of the Labor Party (PT), which extended to other organizations led by the party, such as Central Única dos Trabalhadores CUT (Unified Workers' Central) and its affiliated unions. Besides, the left was weakened in the ideological dispute due to the contradictions in the administrations run by PT, which called themselves left-wing, but demobilized popular organizations, bet on a top-down conciliation strategy and refused to take a class perspective or even to openly challenge more conservative views" (Calil 2020: 77). Setting aside the idealistic tone of the analysis, we generally agree with this critique of PT and affiliated organizations and social movements. However, one must take into consideration the fact that, up until now, there hasn't been any other left-wing alternative capable of swaying social movements in a more radical direction, as the right managed to achieve in its sphere of action. As such, at no point has there been a leftist option that could effectively work to organize the working class aiming towards actual resistance, be it to the coup or to neoliberal policies, beyond PT's electoral and

openly hold far-right opinions. For this reason, the PT's strategy, and Lula's as well, has been to gravitate towards the right in search of alliances with political sectors that participated in the coup but were unhappy with the actions (and inactions) of the current resident of the Planalto Palace.

From a class analysis viewpoint, it is undeniable that the economic and reform policy of the Bolsonaro government pleases the hegemonic sectors, the big bourgeoisie, agribusiness and imperialism. Meanwhile, concessions to the military and to a few selected sectors of the civil service in addition to agreements with (majority) physiological and right-wing sectors of the national congress are trump cards in the dispute for reelection. Even important popular sectors can be seduced by the actions of certain politicians, priests and pastors engaged in the campaign, although the working class, as a whole, having suffered losses as a result of neoliberal policies, the dismantling of previous social policies, the pandemic, unemployment and inflation, and remembering the inclusion process experienced during the 13 years of a PT government, constitutes the main foundation in support of Lula's candidacy.

For the Bolsonaro government seeking reelection keeping its radical middle-class base mobilized is critical, even though this would involve stances that often clash with the desire for political stability and social peace. The lack of a political environment sometimes creates obstacles for the program of neoliberal reform and privatizations. Thus, the government has, from the beginning, been marked by acute tensions that irritate its more pragmatic allies, who would certainly have preferred a more discreet government alternative, one that was not so committed to the so-called "behavioral agenda" and that didn't oppose the scientific consensus.

As we will explain in the next section, the denial approach in relation to the new coronavirus pandemic is an eloquent example of the irrational mindset and actions that seem to characterize the Bolsonaro administration. However, this apparent irrationality does not affect the mainstream neoliberal agreement.[4] In fact, the destructive action of the far-right

---

parliamentary actions, which places the party, and President Lula in particular, as the only effective possibility for the left in today's polarized context.

[4] It is worth highlighting that the apparent irrational acts of the Bolsonaro administration – "a Minister of Communications who undisguisedly emulates Goebbels; a chancellor who believes the country should become an international pariah; a

Brazilian government proved to be quite functional in key moments of the structural (counter)reforms established by Paulo Guedes and Roberto Campos Neto. As Leda Paulani (2021) clarifies, there may appear to be an "innate born incompatibility between Guedes's ultraliberalism and Bolsonaro's despotism. But the affinities between the two sets of beliefs are greater than the inconsistencies propagated by the global and neo-liberal hoax". In other words, the neoliberal project peacefully complies with Jair Bolsonaro's extreme right-wing radicalism, in addition to using the health crisis context as an advantage to swiftly achieve its political and economic goals in Brazil.[5]

Pandemic denial in the Jair Bolsonaro administration

From the beginning of Covid-19 pandemic in Brazil, President Jair Bolsonaro, in tandem with then-president of the United States Donald

---

Minister of Economy that treats the public servant as an enemy […] a Minister of Education that accuses Federal Universities of being drug-ridden places; a Minister of the Environment who remarks that the government should take advantage of the chaos produced by the pandemic in order to pass anti-environmental protection laws under the radar of the press; a Minister of Human Rights who clings to the defense of anti-feminist and religious-fundamentalist agendas; a person in charge of racial equality who announces the discarding of literary-historical collections as it is considered ideologically manipulated; a person responsible for cultural affairs who walks around bearing arms in government facilities […]" (Uchôa 2022: 145) etc. – are acts that notably aim at dismantling the Brazilian State, in line with the dominant radical neoliberalism.

[5] Researcher Pereira Andrade (2020: 8–11), who tries "to understand the *consolidation* of the authoritarian turn of Brazilian neoliberalism," states that the main economic policies proposed by Guedes aiming for large-scale government reform are: (i) pension reform, transitioning from a pay-as-you-go model to a capitalization model; (ii) labor reform, reducing "to the bare minimum companies' labor and pension obligations"; (iii) attacking the ways unions are funded, requiring the payment of the contributions by bank slip; (iv) tax reform, reducing the load on business; (v) taking credit away from the State, permitting state-funded credit only for "microcredit and social programs"; (vi) putting an end to subsidies; (vii) privatizations, proposing "to simply privatize all state-run Brazilian companies"; (viii) proposed constitutional amendment of the federative pact, detaching "public spending, which currently define the percentage of the budget to be spent on education, health, safety, public servant personnel, etc."; (ix) Fiscal Balance plan for states and municipalities, proposing "IMF-style loans" and; (x) radical opening of the economy, cutting import tariffs even more." A significant part of this agenda has already been implemented and the rest is underway, perhaps waiting for Bolsonaro's re-election.

Trump, but at odds with the rest of the world, adopted an openly denialist and anti-scientific position, minimizing the gravity of the situation and delegitimizing the World Health Organization's (WHO) guidelines. He effectively opposed, as part of his political strategy, the social distancing measures, which were adopted and upheld by mayors and governors, when these were, at that point, in which vaccines were still under development, the only way to prevent the dissemination of the virus. Moreover, Bolsonaro engaged in a systematic campaign against the use of masks and defended herd immunity by contagion as well as the use of medications not backed by scientific evidence – which, in turn, encouraged people "to ditch social distancing, creating a false sense of security, representing a [...] political use of the medication [...] by the Brazilian government" (Caponi et al. 2021: 79).[6]

Caponi et al. (2021: 97) employ Achille Mbembe's concept of necropolitics to classify Bolsonaro's apparently irrational attitudes towards the pandemic, insofar as the government "reinforces and reclaims the neoliberal logic centered on the idea of assuming one's own risks and exposing populations to death". It's telling that the government is seeking, essentially, to safeguard businesses' interests in maintaining profit rates, as well as to keep their far-fight ideological base mobilized, spreading the idea that the coronavirus is purportedly a communist creation and that individual freedoms are being impinged by way of social distancing measures and mandatory mask usage. It's worth adding that ministers Paulo Guedes and Ernesto Araújo (of Foreign Affairs) both spouted this anti-scientific, conspiracy-theory narrative, stating that the SARS-CoV-2 came from a Chinese lab, which resulted in diplomatic issues with the Asian giant. In short, necropolitics and science denial are combined and served as fodder to neoliberal discourse itself.

The aim of neoliberalism, especially when it comes to healthcare, was to strengthen private health insurance operators to the detriment of the national unified health service (SUS). This is why the Bolsonaro administration initially nominated Luiz Henrique Mandetta for the Ministry of Health. Mandetta is an orthopedic doctor and a traditional right-wing politician, with deep connections to the interests of private health insurance operators, having even been president of Unimed Campo Grande

---

[6] Researcher Elaine Bortone (2022) has shown how defending medication whose efficacy towards Covid is not backed by scientific evidence was beneficial to several drug companies that support Bolsonaro.

between 2001 and 2004, as well as a vocal critic of the PT administrations' Mais Médicos ("More Doctors") program. It's worth emphasizing that the Mais Médicos program, which was launched in 2013, ensured healthcare to Brazil's poorest citizens, by hiring foreign doctors, especially Cubans, who ended up leaving the country once Bolsonaro was elected in 2018, before he even took office. Bolsonaro had vowed to expel the Cuban doctors and took no effective measure to fill in the gap they had left.

The Covid-19 pandemic, however, forced the minister to get behind SUS, the only way of providing care on a large scale to the sick or to efficiently vaccinate the Brazilian population. Besides, Mandetta did not accept the policy in favor of using demonstrably ineffective medication, with serious side effects, against Covid, which ended up costing him his position as head of the ministry. It also exposed the existence of two alternatives when it came to the problem within the far-right: one being purely neoliberal, but which make concessions, at least momentarily, due to the unforeseen reality of the pandemic, and the other being decidedly necropolitical. Nevertheless, the neoliberal project for the healthcare sector is common to both and had supporters since the early 1990s as a "private health project", which is "diametrically opposite to the project of public health reform" (Bravo, Pelaez and Pinheiro 2018: 11).

After the 2016 coup, the assault on Healthcare and SUS intensified, with a major blow being a reduction in financial resources after the approval of Constitutional Amendment 95, which established the so-called *Teto dos Gastos* ("Spending Cap").[7] According to Santos (2020: 4):

> It's clear that Brazil's misadventure with neoliberalism has earlier chapters, as can be seen with the so-called Law of Fiscal Responsibility, the permission granted to Social Organizations to conduct core State activities and the approval of Law 13.097/15, which allows foreign capital to invest in the country's private healthcare sector. But after the 2016 coup, we have decisively entered a new era of outright "social separation strongly linked to mercantile values, legitimation of inequalities and hate cultures". An era in which "the way democracy operates was altered in itself […] in defense of an autarchization of the exercise of power" (Guimarães and Santos 2019, p. 223).

---

[7] The spending cap rule is an eccentricity implanted by the Temer administration, in which a limit on primary public spending, during a period of 20 years, was inserted in the Magna Carta by way of a constitutional amendment.

A document entitled *Travessia social* ("Social Crossing"), "expressing the social policy of the *Uma Ponte para o Futuro* ['A bridge to the future'] program", presents the main guidelines of the Temer administration against SUS, namely: "an emphasis on managerialism, in which bad management is considered the problem with SUS; the need to focus on the demographic that cannot afford private health insurance; e the stimulus to expand coverage of private insurance" (Bravo, Pelaez and Pinheiro 2018: 13). This project was put into practice by Health Minister Ricardo Barros, whose "campaign for congressman was linked to a private health insurance consortium" and, as head of the Ministry, he introduced as one of the pillars of his administration "a proposal for Low-Income Health Insurance" (Bravo, Pelaez and Pinheiro 2018: 14). However, these lower cost private insurance plans have a number of limitations on medical services, aside from being of low quality, which ultimately requires the public health system to step in to complement the private system's deficiencies (Bravo, Pelaez and Pinheiro 2018).[8]

In the Bolsonaro administration, the privatizing project was introduced initially in both "Paulo Guedes's plan to build a new federative pact," whose aim was the "deconstitutionalization of healthcare spending" (Santos 2020: 1) as well as in Mandetta's proposal to unlink healthcare resources and to "question the gratuity and the universality of SUS, going so far as to state, in an interview, that he would like to take this proposal to Congress" (Alves, Correia and Santos 2021: 74). On the other hand, despite the difference between their respective positions with regard to the Covid-19 response, what is most striking is that the tendency to scale

---

[8] Other connections between the Temer administration and the business sector can be seen in the creation, by way of Instituto Coalizão Brasil (Brazil Coalition Institute), of the document *Coalizão Saúde Brasil: uma agenda para transformar o sistema de saúde (Brazil Health Coalition: an agenda to transform the healthcare system)*, released in 2017: "This document [...] developed by representatives of the health sector supply chain [...] is aimed towards challenging and building a new healthcare system for Brazil [...] The group defends the thesis that the public and private sectors need to build an integrated chain of continuous care [...]. Other measures by the Health Ministry in this administration are proposals for Alterations in the Health Insurance Plan Law. In September 2017, Rogério Marinho (PSDB/RN), the leader of the Special Committee on Health Insurance Plans of the Chamber of Deputies, laid out the main points he hoped to include in his report, which were: Repeal of the Health Insurance Plan Law [...] - Segmentation of Coverage [...] – Readjustment after 60 years of age [...] – Reduction in reimbursement value to SUS" (Bravo, Pelaez and Pinheiro 2018: 16–17).

down the role of the State wasn't interrupted, even after the pandemic started. On the contrary, since the answers provided by the Bolsonaro administration to the public health crises caused by the novel coronavirus went "towards strengthening the commodification of healthcare" (Alves, Correia & Santos 2021: 76), as moves that benefit private healthcare, insurance plans and policies can attest to:

> [...] whether through ways to use public healthcare funds by the private sector, when the State pays the sector for hospital services by renting out hospital beds for patients with Covid-19, even without adopting the practice of single queue access to these beds; or by handing out the management of public services, such as the field hospitals, to the privately-owned Social Health Organizations [OSS - Organizações Sociais de Saúde]. (Alves, Correia and Santos 2021: 82)

It's worth noting that even as the country faced high death rates, the Bolsonaro government, giving continuity to neoliberal healthcare policies, published the controversial Decree 10.530 in October 2020, which "foresaw the privatization of primary care," which would bring about considerable damage to Brazilian society. However, facing "countless pressure from entities, social movements and society at large" (Alves, Correia & Santos2021: 74), the president was forced to withdraw the decree. According to Cislaghi (2021: 21–22):

> The decree qualified the policy to promote the primary health care sector within the scope of the Investment Partnership Program (PPI) for the preparation of studies of alternative partnerships with the private sector to build, modernize and run the Primary Care Units (UBS - Unidades Básicas de Saúde) with the creation of pilot projects. The proposal's negative repercussions made the government retract from the decree, but they promised to deliver an edited version in the following weeks.

The forces leading to the withdrawal of the decree took place in the context of an uncontrolled public health crisis, in which both of the aforementioned positions crossed swords amidst the chaos, with intense debates raging between the Federal Government, governors and mayors, not to mention the Supreme Court, which was frequently called upon to intervene in the case. All of this was closely followed by the corporate media, which was also torn between the two positions. Nevertheless, none of this disturbed the privatizing consensus, although a certain degree of caution prevailed, counter to the administration's position, towards not promoting sudden changes in the context of the pandemic.

After Mandetta was laid off, the post of Health Minister was given to Nelson Teich, an oncologist with ties to corporate interests. However, he quit in less than one month on the job, after being forced to sign a protocol recommending the early employment of medications that are not supported by scientific evidence for mild-to-moderate cases of Covid-19 (Bueno and Ventura 2021). The position was then handed to General Eduardo Pazuello, who didn't have a degree in a health-related field, and who even went so far as admitting, on record, that "before becoming a minister he 'didn't know what SUS was'" (Bueno and Ventura 2021: 452). Strongly aligned with the institutional strategies of scientific denial, the new minister doggedly defended the use of chloroquine and ivermectin, drugs that made up the so-called "Covid Kit". He also created, in the ministry, the web portal TrateCov, which recommended, regardless of symptoms and cases, treatment with an identical list of ineffective medications.

The truth is that Pazuello had already taken on a leadership position in the ministry under Teich's tenure. The argument was that he was a military man specialized in logistics. What his command effectively shows is a far-reaching militarization process within the Health Ministry, emblematic of what is taking place in Bolsonaro's government as a whole, which includes military personnel that lack the necessary technical knowledge to occupy a variety of posts, including those at the top level.[9] Furthermore, not even the alleged competence in logistics was demonstrated, as was attested in the negligence in providing oxygen for the treatment of Covid-19, especially in the emblematic case in the state of Amazonas.

But setting up ministries headed by the military is nothing more than a practice to strengthen neoliberal policies, bringing about a series of complications even beyond the context of the public health crisis, given that militarization contests the republican perspective itself, seeing as "military training is not geared towards democratic conflict management, but by the logic of war" (Silva 2021). In light of the reality of the pandemic, the losses that stem from the militarization of government organs are even greater, especially when the person responsible for healthcare,

---

[9] In the explanation of Bueno and Ventura (2021: 451), "up until the end of the first semester of 2020, 25 director or high-level technical positions in the Ministry of Health had already been occupied by military personnel, of which 21 had no prior experience in the health sector".

operating on a hierarchical dynamic of submission to the president's orders, strictly adheres to an ideological strategy of disease containment through genocidal and anti-scientific policies (Silva 2021). In this way, "Health Ministry's militarization process corresponds to the ideological subjugation of a traditional Brazilian state institution, whose public policies stopped being informed by expertise or by science" (Bueno and Ventura 2021: 456).

The fact is that the neoliberal privatization project, which takes advantage of "historical dismantling produced by definancing […] and by making workers more precarious in order to reduce political resistance to these measures" (Cislaghi 2021: 23), remained strong during the entire Bolsonaro administration. The (fourth) current Health Minister, Marcelo Queiroga, is a cardiologist and, up until his nomination to the ministry, was the managing partner of the company Cardiocenter. The minister, who also tries to diligently follow the negationist directions of the head of state, recently made an announcement, which wasn't met with significant contestation on the part of corporate media, under the pretense of increasing competition between private health insurance providers, the creation of an open system by the name of *open health*. As in the case of open banking, this would be "a repository of health and healthcare data of every Brazilian, collected from an electronic medical chart; and a 'positive record of health,' with financial data on health insurance recipients" (Fraga and Rocha 2022). This initiative seeks to encourage people to leave SUS, allowing private companies "to select patients according to the disease and its severity. That is, to sell cheap policies to healthy people and more expensive policies to those with some type of illness. If they can afford it…" (Castro and Castro 2022).

The following rather long quote from Caponi et al. (2021: 82–83) is important because it emphatically summarizes the connections between scientific denial and the neoliberal project of the Bolsonaro administration and how this connection is putting Brazilian lives at risk:

> Advocates of neoliberalism believe that they will benefit from a smaller State, with less taxes, less investments in education and public health, transformed into spaces for market dispute. It is up to each of us to manage and anticipate risks, pay for health insurance, get a pension, save some capital. When this neoliberal logic bumps up against a dramatic phenomenon such as the Covid-19 pandemic, the frailties of a market-regulated healthcare model stand out. With the onset of the pandemic, many countries started investing heavily in public health, in science and technology. Yet, even in the context

of the precariousness of SUS and the rise in Covid-19 cases and deaths, the Brazilian government employed less than 40% of the budget set aside to fight the pandemic. This underemployment of resources is one of the elements that, along with defending the use of chloroquine, with the critique of social distancing and the mask usage, and the lack of consideration towards purchasing an effective vaccine, sets up a true necropolitical (Mbembe 2011) management of the pandemic, which is not about living and reducing mortality, but about letting people die, systematically exposing citizens to the danger of contagion and of death.

The main international data on Covid-19 and the Brazilian scenario

According to Graph 1, the global ranking for the top ten countries with the highest number of Covid-19 cases, on April 20, 2022, is as follows: the United States (80.80 million), India (43.05 million), Brazil (30.31 million), France (28.03 million), Germany (23.84 million), the United Kingdom (21.96 million), Russia (17.84 million), South Korea (16.67 million), Italy (15.86 million) and Peru (15.01 million). The number of Covid-19 cases by million inhabitants in these same countries, as illustrated in Graph 2, and their respective global rank in the same period is France (415,677 → 18th), South Korea (324,997 → 30th), the United Kingdom (322,010 → 32nd), Germany (284,200 → 40th), Italy (262,698 → 43rd), the United States (242,710 → 51st), Brazil (141,649 → 83rd), Russia (122,252 → 93rd), Peru (106,653 → 98th) and India (30,895 → 143rd).[10]

---

[10] The ranking in the number of Covid-19 cases by million inhabitants begins as follows: Faroe Islands (706,542), Denmark (533,946), Andorra (530,199), Cypress (519,849), Gibraltar (519.248), Iceland (498,115), Slovenia (481,272), Holland (473.067), San Marino (472,684) and Slovakia (460,318).

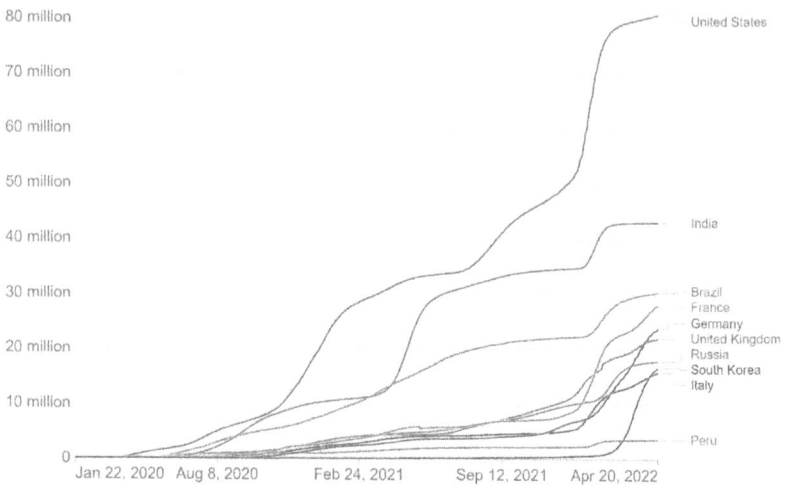

Graph 1 – Global ranking of total number of Covid-19 cases – April 20, 2022.
Source: Our World in Data: https://ourworldindata.org/

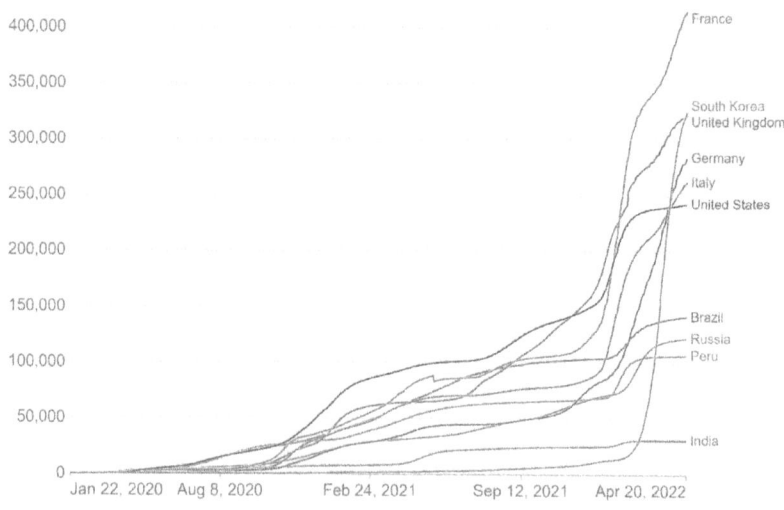

Graph 2 – Number of Covid-19 cases per million inhabitants – April 20, 2022, in select countries.
Source: Our World in Data: https://ourworldindata.org/

Graph 3 illustrates the ranking of the top ten countries with the most deaths due to Covid-19, on April 20, 2022, and they are the United States (990,208), Brazil (662,659), India (522,062), Russia (366,654), Mexico (324,004), Peru (212,704), the United Kingdom (172,551), Italy (162,098), Indonesia (155,937) and France (144,683). When it comes to total deaths by million inhabitants, as seen in graph 4, these same countries have the following numbers and positions on the ranking, respectively: Peru (6,376 → 1st), Brazil (3,097 → 15th), the United States (2,974 → 20th), Italy (2,685 → 28th), the United Kingdom (2,530 → 31st), Russia (2,513 → 33rd), Mexico (2,487 → 34th), France (2,146 → 43rd), Indonesia (564 → 117th) and India (378 → 131st).[11]

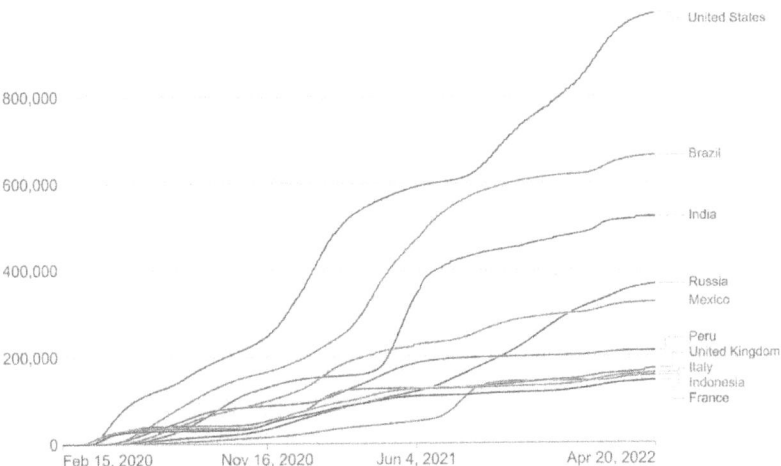

Graph 3 – Global ranking in total deaths due to Covid-19 – April 20, 2022.
Source: Our World in Data: https://ourworldindata.org/

---

[11] The global ranking of the ten countries with the most deaths associated to Covid-19 by million inhabitants, corresponding to available data from the same period, is as follows: Peru (6,376), Bulgaria (5,340), Bosnia and Herzegovina (4,827), Hungary (4,775), North Macedonia (4,449), Montenegro (4,315), Georgia (4,220), Croatia (3,860), Czech Republic (3,733) and Slovakia (3,632).

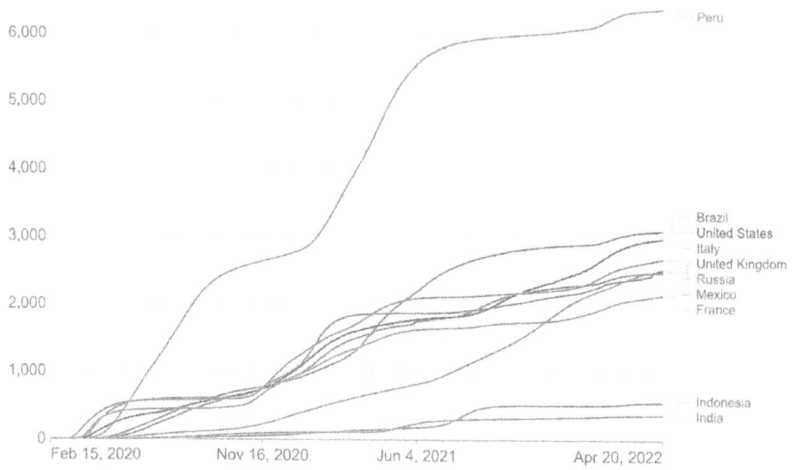

Graph 4 – Number of Covid-19 deaths per million inhabitants – April 20, 2022, in select countries.
Source: Our World in Data: https://ourworldindata.org/

By way of conclusion: Vaccines and subservience

In conclusion, it's worth underscoring, once more, how the Bolsonaro administration transformed the pandemic crisis into a political dispute battlefield and how only after the individual states were close to conducting their own vaccination campaigns, especially the state of São Paulo, which had developed the CoronaVac vaccine, did the Federal Government finally buy the first doses of the vaccine, even though they did not have an application schedule laid out yet, which proves that the measure was not being planned. Furthermore, even with vaccination measures in place and despite the vaccine's high acceptance by the Brazilian population, Bolsonaro continued betting on a narrative war, defending the so-called early treatment and spreading fake news concerning the efficacy and side effects of the vaccines, especially in children.[12]

---

[12] Hastily, and in opposition to WHO guidelines, but in line with Bolsonaro's re-election strategies, Health Minister Marcelo Queiroga announced the end of the Public Health Emergency of National Concern in Brazil on April 22. After this point, a variety of exceptional measures to fight the virus ceased to be valid and private corporations received authorization to sell Covid-19 vaccines without conditional donations of doses to SUS (Lopes 2022).

It must also be said that the Parliamentary Commission of Inquiry (CPI), installed in the Senate on April 27th 2021, had an important role in investigating and recording President Bolsonaro's denialism and obscurantism, not to mention in instigating the Federal Government to take some action to handle the pandemic. The two major lines of investigation were: "[i] the adoption of the herd immunity strategy adopted by the Bolsonaro's government and its allegedly 'parallel cabinet' to combat the pandemic, [ii] and the supposed corruption and prevarication infraction on hospital utensils and vaccines acquisition by the government and private companies" (Alves, Oliveira & Silva 2021: 81–82).

Among other issues that are expressed in the inquiry's robust final report, what was found is that the Bolsonaro administration (a) repeatedly refused initial offerings of the vaccine from the company Pfizer, which had its eye on the sizeable Brazilian market and on the country's historically successful vaccination campaigns, given the renowned technical and organizational capabilities of SUS, (b) decided to purchase only the lowest possible quota of vaccines offered by the international consortium Covax Facility and (c) agreed to the corruption scheme engendered in the acquisition process of the Covaxin vaccine, from Indian biotech company Bharat Biotech. As well as (d) promoting a systematic campaign against vaccines, especially CoronaVac, developed using Chinese technology by the Butantã Institute, a public institution tied to the state of São Paulo, and (e) not coming up with any effective action to viably produce a national vaccine, keeping in mind the country had the capacity to do so, which would require financial resources, organization and institution support of Public Universities, which, on the contrary, throughout the entire administration have suffered radical budget cuts and political interference, including the nomination of intervening deans.[13]

---

[13] Based on evidence produced during the five months of inquiry, the CPI indicted several political agents, public servants and private companies that deliberately did not make the decisions that needed to be made or were connected with criminal actions. In short, the CPI "[...] indicted 65 people and 2 private companies, Prevent Senior [medical group] and VTC logistics company. Among those investigated are the last and the current Minister of Health, Eduardo Pazuello and Marcelo Queiroga, respectively; the former Minister of Foreign Affairs, Ernesto Araújo; the former advisor of the Presidency, Arthur Weintraub; two of Bolsonaro's sons, Congressman Eduardo Bolsonaro and Senator Flávio Bolsonaro; and the President Jair Bolsonaro himself. The crimes attributed to the President totalized 29 types such as epidemy crime; quackery; sanitary measure violation; active corruption; fraudulent misrepresentation;

There is another aspect of the problem worth highlighting, one which illustrates the position of the Bolsonaro administration, breaking with traditional positions on the matter in the country. According to Daibert et al. (2022: 88), there is a vaccine apartheid, meaning that, whereas in the central countries "the challenges involve increasing confidence in the vaccine, combatting fake news and the politicization of the vaccine", in the African continent, vaccine scarcity "doesn't even allow for health professionals to be vaccinated". This fact is fundamentally the result of the patent system, whose main goal is the profitability of the extremely concentrated oligopoly of the global pharmaceutical industry, relegating to the background the protection of a large part of the world's population. In this context, in October 2020, the governments of South Africa and India markedly asked the World Trade Organization (WTO) to suspend intellectual property related to Covid-19 treatments.[14]

Although the patent waiver agreement would provide an increase in the global vaccine supply, allowing for a global response to the circulating SARS-Cov-2 virus and to the new variants, "the idea was back by approximately one hundred developing countries, but could not counter the position of the richest nations in the world" (Marques 2022: 1688). Brazil was one of the only so-called developing nations that stood against the suspension of the patents, seeing as the Bolsonaro administration always subserviently followed in the footsteps of the Trump administration. However, the American president changed his mind at the end of

---

inciting to crime; private documents fraud; irregular employment of public funds; prevarication; crimes against humanity as extermination, persecution, and inhumane acts to cause intentional suffering; and liability crimes" (Alves, Oliveira and Silva 2021: 82–83).

[14] One aspect of the vaccine inequality is well explained by Marques (2022: 1689) using data: "According to a study from Duke's Global Health Innovation Center, developed countries, which represent one fifth of the world's population, bought around 6 billion doses; whereas less developed and developing nations only guaranteed around 2,6 billion doses. This amount includes the 1.1 billion doses attributed to Covax, an arrangement in which international financiers committed to vaccinating one fifth of the global population. Through this mechanism, investigators claim, it could take two years or more until the entire population of less developed countries is fully immunized." The Covax Facility consortium is an international fund coordinated by the WHO and Gavi (Global Alliance for Vaccines and Immunization) to purchase and distribute vaccines to so-called developing countries. However, as Daibert et al. (2022: 88) explain, the Covax mechanism "is seen as a futile promise that failed in equitably distributing the vaccines, as well as not involving civil society and low-income countries in a structured way".

his administration, which in turn made the Brazilian government more flexible in their position, even though it did not go on to support South Africa and India's correct initiative (Chade 2022). The fact is that around a year and a half after the waiver request, the matter has not yet been defined; there's only a sign of an initial understanding between the main countries in the WHO, with the caveat that "for activists, the proposal should not even be called a 'patent waiver agreement,' given the imposed demands, which will make the deal pointless" (ibid.).

Bibliography

Alves, Gleisse, Fernanda Oliveira and Letícia Silva (2021). "Parliamentary Inquiry Committee (CPI) on Covid-19 pandemic in Brazil and the defense of democracy in crisis", in *A crise da Covid-19 no Brasil e seus reflexos*, Alves, Gleisse et al. (ed.), Brasília: CEUB, 73–84.

Alves, Pâmela, Correia, Maria and Santos, Viviane (2021). "A mercantilização da saúde no enfrentamento da covid-19: o fortalecimento do Setor privado", in *Revista Humanidades e Inovação*, 35 (8), 71–85.

Bolaño, César, Cabral Filho and Adilson Vaz (2014), "O Brasil e o movimento social global: uma análise dos eventos de junho de 2013 em perspectiva histórica", in *Liinc Em Revista*, 1 (10), 10–21.

Bolaño, César and Zanghelini, Fabrício (2022). "Reforma Trabalhista de 2017: a ampliação da exploração da força de trabalho em meio ao avanço das políticas neoliberais", in *Crítica y Resistencias*, 14, 204–223.

Bortone, Eliane de Almeida (2022). "O governo Jair Bolsonaro e os empresários da indústria farmacêutica", in *Marx e o Marxismo*, 17 (9), 246–270.

Bravo, Maria, Pelaez, Elaine and Pinheiro, Wladimir (2018). "As contrarreformas na política de saúde do governo Temer", in *Argum*, 1 (10), 9–23.

Bueno, Flávia and Ventura, Deisy (2021). "De líder a paria de la salud global: Brasil como laboratorio del 'neoliberalismo epidemiológico' ante la Covid-19", in *Foro Internacional*, 2 (LXI), 427–467.

Calil, Gilberto (2020). "Brasil: o negacionismo da pandemia como estratégia de fascistização", in *Materialismo Storico*, 2 (IX).

Caponi, Sandra et al. (2021). "O uso político da cloroquina: COVID-19, negacionismo e neoliberalismo", in *Revista brasileira de sociologia*, 21 (9), 78–102.

Castro, Ana and Castro, Cosette (2022). "A quem interessa o Open Health?", in *Correio Braziliense*. <https://blogs.correiobraziliense.com.br/coletivo-filhas-da-mae/2022/01/31/a-quem-interessa-o-open-health/>.

Chade, Jamil (2022). "Acordo mundial de patentes de vacinas contra covid exclui Brasil", in *Uol*. <https://noticias.uol.com.br/colunas/jamil-chade/2022/03/17/acordo-de-patentes-de-vacinas-contra-covid-exclui-brasil.htm>.

Cislaghi, Juliana (2021). "Financiamento e privatização da saúde no brasil em tempos ultraneoliberais", in *Revista Humanidades e Inovação*, 35 (8), 15–24.

Daibert, Lara et al. (2022). "Mais de um ano após o início da vacinação, a exigência de equidade na distribuição de vacinas é destaque nas manifestações da sociedade civil", in *Cadernos CRIS/FIOCRUZ sobre saúde global e diplomacia da saúde*, 2, 84–89.

Demier, Felipe (2015), "Nas ruas por direitos: uma análise das jornadas de junho de 2013", in *Esquerda Online*. <https://esquerdaonline.com.br/2015/01/16/nas-ruas-por-direitos-uma-analise-das-jornadas-de-junho-de-2013/>.

Finguerut, Ariel and Souza, Marco Aurélio Dias de (2018). "Que Direita é Esta? As Referências a Trump na Nova Direita Brasileira Pós-Michel Temer", in *Revista TOMO*, 33, 229–269.

Fraga, Armínio and Rocha, Rudi (2022). "Por que o 'open helth'?", in *Folha de São Paulo*. <https://www1.folha.uol.com.br/opiniao/2022/03/por-que-o-open-health.shtml>.

Guimarães, J and Santos, Ronaldo T, (2019) "Em busca do tempo perdido: anotações sobre os determinantes políticos da crise do SUS". *Saúde em Debate*, v.43, pp. 219-233.

Lopes, Raquel (2022). "Vacinas contra Covid começam a ser vendidas a clínicas privadas em maio no Brasil", in *Folha de São Paulo*. < https://www1.folha.uol.com.br/equilibrioesaude/2022/04/vacinas-contra-covid-comecam-a-ser-vendidas-a-clinicas-privadas-em-maio-no-brasil.shtml>.

Machado, Jorge and Miskolci, Richard (2019). "Das jornadas de junho à cruzada moral: o papel das redes sociais na polarização política brasileira", in *Sociologia & Antropologia*, 3 (9), 945–970.

Marques, Inês (2022). "A (des)razoabilidade da concessão de patentes em face da proteção da saúde pública?", in *Revista Jurídica Luso-Brasileira*, 2, 1663–1706.

Paulani, Leda (2021). "Dois anos de desgoverno – três vezes destruição", in *A terra é redonda*. <https://aterraeredonda.com.br/dois-anos-de-desgoverno-tres-vezes-destruicao/>.

Pereira Andrade, Daniel (2020). "Neoliberalismo autoritário no Brasil Reforma econômica neoliberal e militarização da administração pública", in *Sens Public*, 1–28.

Santos, Ronaldo Teodoro dos (2020). "O neoliberalismo como linguagem política da pandemia: a Saúde Coletiva e a resposta aos impactos sociais", in *Physis*, 2 (30), 1–9.

Silva, Julia Almeida da (2021). "A militarização do Ministério da saúde e a 'missão cumprida' de Pazuello", in *Le Monde Diplomatique Brasil*. <https://diplomatique.org.br/a-militarizacao-do-ministerio-da-saude-e-a-missao-cumprida-de-pazuello/>.

Soares, Raquel (2018). "Governo Temer e contrarreforma na política de saúde: a inviabilização do SUS", in *Argumentum*, 1 (10), 24–32.

Souza, Jessé de (2014). "A cegueira do debate brasileiro sobre as classes sociais", in *Interesse Nacional*, 27, 35–47.

Uchôa, Marcelo (2022). "Lava Jato: guerra híbrida, lawfare e ataque à democracia no Brasil", in *Sul Global*, 1 (3), 137–151.

Health crises in images: Possible approximations between three major epidemics in Brazil

MARCELA BARBOSA LINS – *Universidade Federal de Minas Gerais*
CAIO DAYRELL SANTOS – *Universidade Federal de Minas Gerais*
ÂNGELA CRISTINA SALGUEIRO MARQUES – *Universidade Federal de Minas Gerais*

Introduction

The word "epidemic", from the Greek "epi" (upon or above) and "demos" (people), refers to something that is above or affects populations: contagious manifestations of collective onset. As the etymology suggests, disease outbreaks are inseparable from the people they afflict, allowing to reflect on their subjection to power and their conditions of emergence.

In this chapter, we investigate and compare how the illness involved in three major epidemic episodes manifests itself visually, namely: the yellow fever outbreak from the late 19th century to the early 20th century, the Spanish flu and the Covid-19. More precisely, we present an imagery analysis based on the historical and iconographic archive from Oswaldo Cruz Institute, a research institution linked to the Ministry of Health, and contemporary documentary images, extracted from the documentary film "Estamos te esperando em casa" (We are waiting for you at home), by Cecilia da Fonte and Marcelo Pedroso.

Importantly, both yellow fever and Spanish flu outbreaks were large-scale public health issues – when yellow fever became a nationwide health issue in 1849, this culminated in the creation of the "Junta Central de Higiene" (Central Board of Hygiene), a bureaucratic Imperial body responsible for addressing public health issues. An important milestone within a governmental paradigm aligned with a certain conception of hygiene and management of population health and life (Rego, 2020

[1851]). The Spanish flu, the largest pandemic of the 20th century, increased the average mortality rate by 2,000 % (Goulart, 2005). Covid-19, in turn, totals 675,000 deaths[1] and points to a management marked by multiple antagonisms, conspiracy theories and denialism.

Montage and framings: A biopolitical visual analysis

In his famous essay, "Images in Spite of All", Georges Didi-Huberman says that "we often ask too much or too little of the image" (2012 [2004]: 32). Many times, we are often tempted to demand that they offer us undeniable proof of a past event as if they could authenticate an objective fact by themselves. Of course, this approach leads to frustration as an image can never show us "the whole truth". This does not mean though that they should be ignored. Images shouldn't be taken as simple "simulacra", an untrustworthy reproduction of reality only suited at most to illustrate. Images, to Didi-Huberman, are an exceptional source of knowledge that scholars cannot take the luxury to neglect.

In his quest to assert the epistemological prominence of images, Didi-Huberman (2011, 2012 [2004]) uses as a methodological reference the "Mnemosyne Atlas" project, produced in 1928 and 1929 by the German art historian Aby Warburg. Named after the Greek muse of memory, the project consisted of a set of dozens of panels, altogether containing around a thousand images, including reproductions of works of art, photographs, documents and parts of books that were enumerated and assembled from a certain subject. The boards involved the most varied themes, from science, religion and pagan practices; from representations of epic scenes to everyday objects; from old traditions to early trends; and from the sophisticated to the ordinary (Müller, 2018).

As the images were not fixed, Warburg could assemble, disassemble and reassemble them as many times as he wanted, thus comparing heterogeneous elements, juxtaposing images taken from different sources and performing procedures such as grouping and regrouping, placing and shifting, and cropping and amplifying details. Each montage and reassembly weaves a nexus from associations, clashes or tensions between images that, in turn, summons a new visual elaboration. The atlas can

---

[1] Available at: https://covid19.who.int/. Access on August 21, 2022.

never be finalized. Its organization is always provisional and incomplete; therefore, it is a "knowledge-movement" (Didi-Huberman, 2013.

The "motor" of this process would be the imagination. He recognizes that this word may sound overindulgent, but it is nonetheless a practice strongly committed to a form of empiricism. The montage, according to Didi-Huberman, is "the activity where the imagination becomes a technique". Photographs, films and other visual archives are always incomplete and have to be placed next to other images, documents and testimonies. By looking between these sets of fragments, the historian is able to make sense of the assemblages and speculate on some missing links without downplaying its own uncertainties. According to Georges Didi-Huberman (2019 [2009]), montage refers to a "network of relations (…) hidden behind events [for] no matter what happens, there is always another reality behind that which is described" (2019 [2009]: 55). As Schwarte (2018) remarked:

> This process of restitution does not claim to say what these images actually show: but, in a more elementary manner, it retraces the circumstances, the dangers, the conditions of possibility of these photographs, along their path through the different stages of production, dissimulation, transmission, manipulation and retouching. This act of restitution displays them as fragments of a particular despair, revolt, organized resistance, defeat and survival. (Schwarte & Woodall, 2018: 81)

Taking the Atlas as inspiration, Didi-Huberman (2019 [2009]: 19–20) sees the montage as "an instrument not for the logical exhaustion of given possibilities, but for the inexhaustible opening to possibilities not yet given". It is, in this way, a way of assembling and disassembling history via framing and intervals. A moving territory which heuristically multiplies the viewpoints – as opposed to the historicity of the empty and homogeneous time, to which Walter Benjaminrefers. In other words, the objective is not to resort to images to categorize or summarize reality but, through a free and holistic exercise, to take them as entry points from where we can figure out larger processes, events and social relations, conjunctions of actors and practices, structures, and technologies. Although the montage method does not pretend to arrive at a definitive thesis or to even follow a fixed procedure, it allows us to highlight hidden links and produce unprecedented associations, dispensing any previous script to do so. To sum up, montage is about disposing objects with the intent to expose relations between them.

This approach is not without risks though. W. J. T. Mitchell (2016) comments on how Warburg seems to think of the work of the historian as a kind of forensics, in which they should investigate the images of the past in a similar fashion as a policeperson looks for pieces of evidence in a crime scene. By making connections between things that are at first glance unrelated, the montage is able to read what was never written. Even so, Mitchell notices that in popular culture there are many improvised wall atlas, an especially common trope in crime and spy thrillers, in which the investigator pins up and plots out all their clues in trying to solve the mystery. Nonetheless, he also points out that these walls of chipboard, newspaper cuttings, photographs and maps are also equally common to conspiracist theorists, whose paranoia leads them to see hidden patterns everywhere. The montage inherently walks a fine line between "method" and "madness", in which you can never truly know if you are finding something truly new or just inferring a pre-established assumption in a random set of pictures.

The montage, as any scholastic work, is not exempt from biases; however, Mitchell might underestimate Warburg and Didi-Huberman's commitment to the gaps and openings of the images: "The patterns that conspiracy theorists discern in everything […] are never dialectical. They assimilate everything into one, non-dialectical pattern" (De Cauwer, 2018: 138). As we wrote before, this kind of visual analysis presupposes that an image does not contain any truth by itself; therefore, it is not suitable to prove anything. The montage, in this sense, has fewer parallels to police work and more to what Eyal Weizman (2014) conceives as forensis, the etymological origin for "forensics" which means "pertaining to the forum". Instead of confirming or demonstrating a specific stance on something, the montage assembles several images with the intent of creating a public and political open discussion about a subject and avoiding any fixed stances.

Thinking about possible rapprochements between the Spanish flu, yellow fever and Covid-19 in Brazil spurred us to seek juxtapositions that would highlight overt biopolitical framings, especially in three regimes of visuality which guide our gaze and interpretations when we stand among the selected images. At first, we tried to bring together images that somehow produced certain bodiliness marked by removal of agency, suffering and disappearance of the way of life which guided people's experience until then. In these images, we identified framings that pointed to the production of suffering bodies and of bodies qualified to combat suffering. Next, we showed that despite the predominance of biopolitical framings of control, containment, annihilation and destruction which defined human and non-human actions during epidemics, some fractures gave glimpses into the power of affections, embracement, bonds and resources that redefine the conditions of vulnerability and the agency scope of subjects.

Hence, the images are experienced as anachronism exercises, in which multiple temporalities are juxtaposed to bring about a critical regard in history. In other words, montage dismantles our habitual perception of relationships and, by distancing it, creates new groupings between orders of reality (Huberman, 2009). In light of this, the analyses presented here will be articulated based on a gaze that both situates the images in history – at their time of production – and proposes new articulations and relations between the presented temporalities.

Drawing from Georges Didi-Huberman (2017 [2009]), Jacques Rancière (2017, 2018, 2019, 2021) and Judith Butler (2015 [2009], 2017 [2012], 2019 [2014]), we explore aspects of image politics and their relations with ethical dimensions of human dignity. We ask ourselves whether the imagery representation that reproduces framings of ill subjects lacking agency exposes them to oblivion or if, somehow, these images could offer clues, even if minor, of gestures proper to a political appearance. We believe that reflecting on how images from the three epidemics juxtapose and intersect can stem from understanding how they result from choices that place photographers, photographs and spectators in relationships guided by specific frames. To us, montage, this aesthetic and political gesture of approaching and articulating (through clashes) images belonging to different historical regimes, can help us identify continuities and ruptures in the "dispositifs" that guide ways of life and the possibilities of their experiences.

In "Precarious Life", Butler (2019 [2014]) indicates what the conditions are for elaborating a framing of the living conditions of vulnerable populations, showing concern for how situations of flagrant threat and disrespect for basic survival needs and human dignity are framed to conceal, or at least disguise, the arbitrary elements of power that exists at the heart of such situations. Visibility of precarious life, when built from control frames mostly produced and legitimized by the state, creates interpretative schemes which tend to highlight suffering and death scenarios as commonplace. Such operations, according to Butler, help define which lives are grievable: so when we speak about frames in this respect, we are not simply talking about theoretical perspectives that we bring to the analysis of politics but about modes of intelligibility that further the workings of the state and, as such, are themselves exercises of power even as they exceed the specific domain of state power (Butler, 2015 [2009]: 213).

The practical exercise of juxtaposing heterogeneous images in which an entire population is under threat of death can help us get to know the terms, conventions and general norms involved in the production of framings which define regimes of visibility and intelligibility capable of shaping an individual into a recognizable subject. These categories and norms prepare and establish a subject for recognition, which induce such a subject, precede and make recognizability possible. "We cannot easily recognize life outside the frames in which it is given, and those frames not only structure how we come to know and identify life but constitute sustaining conditions for those very lives" (Butler, 2015 [2009]: 44).

The suffering body and its isolation: Barriers imposed on mobility and sharing

Images construe representations in which the sick body is depicted as suffering, precarious and lacking agency, often in line with historically construed colonial and hierarchical ideologies. Technical devices and apparatus appear in images of the three epidemics analysed to better contain the sick body, isolating it from all structures that articulated its previous life. The forms of containment and extraction of bodies from the shared world were accompanied by governmental measures aimed at controlling the breathing of bodies and silencing any other possibility of action during epidemics. Inhospitality prevailed in the extraction of contaminated bodies from their contexts, under frames of threat and revulsion. Moreover, these images configure a certain commitment to accommodate the spectator into a position of pity and judgement separate from the lives depicted there. Furnished with various equipment, the places intended for treating the ill trigger an image in which the suffering body is pierced, invaded, sedated and "packed" (let us recall how a body with Covid-19 is wrapped in several layers of plastic film for burial) by medical practices.

Health crises in images: three epidemics in Brazil

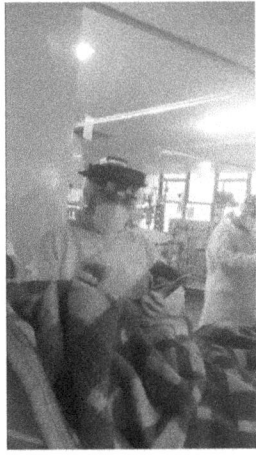

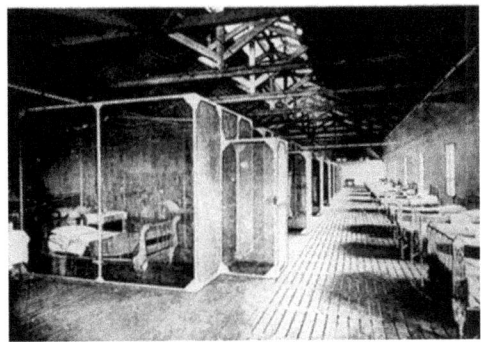

Figure 1. Frame of 'Estamos te esperando em casa'.

Figure 2. Insulated rooms for isolation of yellow fever patients.

The spatialities in which bodies suffer reveal the state of emergency-driving framings of action during epidemics: mobility is halted, freedom of access is restricted, everyday life is frayed and public space vitality is undermined.

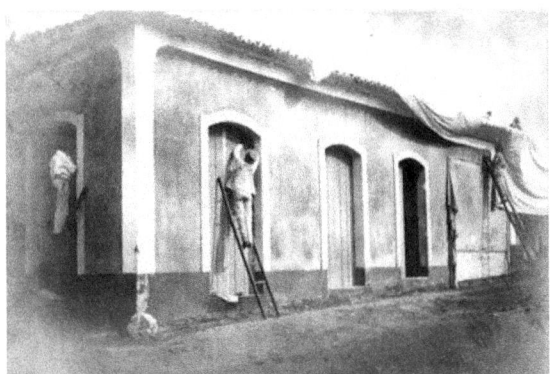

Figure 3. Isolation of a house infected by the yellow fever mosquito, 1905.

During a state of emergency, images reveal how the virus "invasion" transforms safe spaces of affection into war zones, transforms homes into a place of danger and contamination. The image above depicts the Yellow Fever Prophylaxis Service's action during the outbreak in Rio de Janeiro in 1905, a moment in which crisis management was strongly tied to actions not only on the city's topography but also on individual bodies. In the photograph, we see health agents sealing an infected home with canvas and wood, alluding to quarantine measures, recurrent since the successive bubonic plague epidemics in 14th-century Asia and Europe (Santos, 2021). Homes were often sealed during the successive outbreaks of yellow fever, and lazarettos – a quarantine station for the ill – such as the one at Ilha do Bom Jesus, were created in Rio de Janeiro (Rego, 2020 [1851]).

Importantly, the management of yellow fever was closely related to the changes in urban topography, especially due to the influence of anti-contagion theories. In general, this postulate drew attention to and promoted programmes to remove elements considered to spread epidemic diseases: garbage, sewage, polluted water, and overcrowded and poorly ventilated dwellings. According to Roberto Machado (1978: 246), the outbreak was responsible for the new orientation given to public hygiene in Brazil; as mentioned, this was a violent epidemic, whose first cases appeared in December 1849 and spread across several coastal cities. Although it was not the first outbreak to hit the country, it was the first to reach such large proportions.

Despite existing hygiene measures, there was no centralized government body focused on population health management. The Ministry of the Empire thus takes over health during the yellow fever outbreak, asking for support from the Imperial Academy of Medicine,[2] which elaborated a plan to combat the epidemic. Entitled "Providências para prevenir e atalhar o progresso de febre amarela, mandadas executar pelo Ministério por aviso desta data" [Measures to prevent and curb the spread of yellow fever, ordered by the Ministry by notice of this date], the 1850 document presented a detailed plan to combat the pathogen, focused on control over individuals and city life. As Machado sates, "faced with the not only possible but active danger, hygienic measures are exacerbated to such a degree that all life in the city is organized to destroy the epidemic disease" (Machado, 1978: 244).

---

[2] Founded in 1835, the Imperial Academy of Medicine was a body derived from the Medicine Society of Rio de Janeiro, an institution created in 1829 by some physicians who constituted the Brazilian medical elite, following Brazil's independence.

Among the measures put into practice were (1) the creation of an agency dedicated to public health issues; (2) urban planning measures; (3) institution of free care services to impoverished populations; (4) sanitary inspection services conducted periodically in ships, markets, prisons, hospitals, etc., and (5) inspection of the exercise of medicine, surgery and pharmacy. From this model is born the Public Hygiene Board, an organ then linked to the imperial bureaucracy, which was later replaced by the General Inspectorate of Hygiene in 1890. However, despite the centralization efforts, population health care remained mostly the responsibility of the states and municipalities (Hochman, 2011 [1998]).

In practical terms, beyond the institution of a managing body focused on public health issues, we notice a management that pointed to a supposed relationship between certain ways of life and illness. In a statement published by Diário do Rio de Janeiro,[3] the "visit" of yellow fever is signified as a result of the "miserable sanitary state" of the capital's streets. Another statement, published by the same newspaper,[4] exposed the Empire's guidelines for the populations, which are as follows: remove oneself from the city and move to "high and salubrious" places, take extra care with grooming, and live in spacious places with plenty of natural light.

Collective housing was perceived as epidemic irradiation foci, besides being fertile ground for the spread of vices (Chalhoub, 2018 [1996]). In practical terms, this took place with the implementation of a series of urban reforms that culminated, for example, in the demolition of Cabeça de Porco, the most notorious tenement house in Rio de Janeiro, which once housed 4,000 people – an act conducted in line with the normalization of urban space, envisioned to insert the city into a modern paradigm of urbanization.

During the Spanish flu epidemic, in turn, we collected several images that show physicians and their nursing teams visiting the outskirts of Rio de Janeiro. Taking place between 1918 and 1919, management of the disease was linked not to transformations in urban topography but to the institution of mainly non-pharmaceutical measures, namely: the use of medication to alleviate symptoms and measures to control the

---

[3] Diário do Rio de Janeiro, January 30, 1850: 2.
[4] Diário do Rio de Janeiro, February 14, 1850: 1.

displacement of bodies – such as the suspension of non-essential activities (Schwarcz & Starling, 2020).

The following reproductions (Figure. 4 and Figure. 5) show the visits made by physician Arthur Moncorvo Filho in Rio de Janeiro. Moncorvo Filho founded the Institute for Instituto de Proteção e Assistência à Infância (Institute for the Protection and Care to Childhood – IPAI), a private institute of "scientific philanthropy" (Freire & Leony, 2011), which provided services to the population in temporary health units and visits to the outskirts, with partial support from the federal government.

In this context, we call attention to the fact that the Spanish flu epidemic occurs at a time when Brazil was prospecting its institution as a Nation-State, a process that culminated in 1930, with the end of the First Republic. As Gilberto Hochman (2011 [1998]) and Castro-Santos (1985) point out, the first years of the 20th century constitute the historical moment when health becomes not only public but also a state and nationwide issue. This is when we notice an important growth in state activism regarding health and sanitation – which reveals public awareness and governmental responsibility with the country's sanitary conditions and with population health (Hochman, 2011 [1998]).

Thus, philanthropic actions – such as the one undertaken by Moncorvo Filho – were articulated with a broader development process of the sanitary movement in Brazil. It was something overdetermined by the modernization and urbanization process taking place at that time in several regions of the country. As Hochman argues, this is a time when the transition to an urban, industrial society enhanced the problems of mutual dependence. In his words: "promoted a gradual abandonment of both individual […] and voluntary solutions, due to their ineffectiveness before the extent of the problem" (Hochman, 2011 [1998]: 27).

Consequently, biopolitical technologies of population normalization emerged for the then-necessary administration, control and remediation of populations during modernization. The new population density, resulting from the urbanization and industrialization processes, associated with new migratory flows, created previously unknown adversities. Increasing flows between "healthy" and "sick" have intensified and amplified the effects of individual adversities, to the point that "it has become almost impossible to simply isolate oneself from the threats of urban life, for example, through spatial segregation or excluding others from the benefits of services subject to private contract, such as garbage collection and water supply" (Hochman, 2011 [1998]: 29). This points to the fact that health, or disease, is an important example of human interdependence and its solutions.

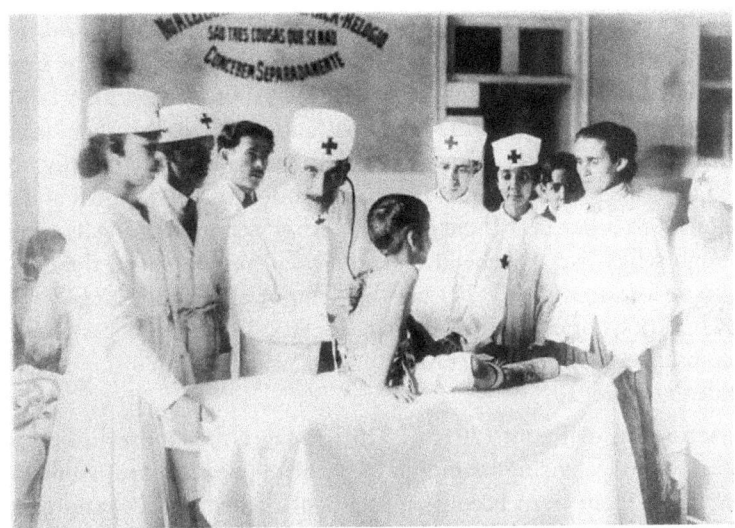

Figure 4. Moncorvo Filho examines a child with pneumonia.

Going back to the images, the backyards once spaces for rest and recovery show sick bodies in stages qualified in the captions as "very serious". Quarantine in domestic spaces and the way infected homes were carefully "packed" make us question which concept of health is at stake in these framings – when the web that preserves their humanity is undone, cutting social bonds and emptying any attempt at sharing and community. Suffering bodies wither amidst power relations that produce and legitimize certain framings, revealing stigmas, prejudices and contempt for certain ways of life and subject positions.

Gazeta de Notícias covered Moncorvo Filho's intervention in Morro do Salgueiro, publishing a news article entitled "A salvação do Morro do Salgueiro" [Morro do Salgueiro's Savior], on 4 November 1918, from which we highlight the following excerpt:

> From the arrival of the entourage at the top of the *morro*, where a veritable multitude of ragged and malnourished creatures surrounded them,

extending their bare hands in supplication, to the extreme misery of the unhygienic pigsties, where illness, hunger, nakedness and death reign, left all with the saddest impression. (Gazeta de Notícias, November 4, 1918: 3)

The text reiterates a frame that exposes the body and bodiliness in their waning, exacerbating the suffering shown through the weakening body. This aspect of how framings produce stigmas is discussed by Erving Goffman and seems to be of particular interest to Butler (2015 [2009], 2019 [2014]), for whom the relational and material web that sustains and defines our degree of exposure to precariousness is directly shattered by how framings affect us and guide our moral judgement and our responses to injustices. Therefore, the author defines framing as "frames through which we apprehend or, indeed, fail to apprehend the lives of others as lost or injured" (2015: 14). Such power relations interfere with the conditions of emergence and consideration of subjects because they circumscribe specific mechanisms through which a way of life is apprehended and judged.

According to Fassin (2016 [2015]), images that individualize pain instead of collectivizing it amplify the control over the most vulnerable, preventing them from becoming agents of their discourses and experiences. Subjects suffering in isolation, having severed all ties with social life, lack humanity and face (demand addressed to the other), which hinders the creation of a collective ethical responsibility based on hospitality, listening and a collective response for those suffering.

Butler therefore questions how widely circulated images are used for a war that oppresses Otherness, personalizing terror, tyranny, villainy or kindness, empathy and hospitality. For them, the images themselves do not define who can or cannot be humanized, as they often present us with "the human face in its deformity and extremity, not the one with which you are asked to identify" (Butler, 2019 [2014]: 126). Our senses are affected by images that control our perceptions and guide our judgements so that we judge the other based on implicit criteria. Thus, questioning the framings involves "a struggle over the domain of appearance and the senses, asking how best to organize media in order to overcome the differential ways through which grievability is allocated" (Butler, 2015 [2009]: 255).

From this perspective, we emphasize that montage, by allowing to juxtapose heterogeneous scenes, helps us to frame the framing, to think its operability and fractures. At the same time, and if "there is no life and no death without a relation to some frame" (Butler, 2015 [2009]: 22), we may better understand how interpretive schemes that "not only structure how we come to know and identify them but constitute their sustaining and legitimizing conditions" work (idem).

Poses staging caring and ailing subjects and the paradigm of progress

Among the selected frames are those in which medical teams appear posing for portraits, following a previously defined script aimed at advertising the successes of the medical team in promoting adequate treatments, highlighting care and aid actions to those considered most vulnerable.

Moncorvo Filho and his team are depicted in a series of staged photos, in which everyone looks at the camera and attests to being part of rescue dispositifs. But the frames produced to document medical teams in their workplaces and the ill suffering often constitute a symbolic violence to the dignity of subjects and groups, forcing them to the immobility of the imposed pose, the lack of autonomy, and the erasure of their unique experiences and trajectories. According to Butler (2019 [2014]), erasure materializes itself through representation, that is, in the context of a dehumanizing representation or when representation captures the Other by simply recognizing an imposed identity. In the case of those marked as ailing subjects, the vulnerability of the body is usually listed as a central, defining and irreversible element which disallows any possibility of action, resistance or transformation.

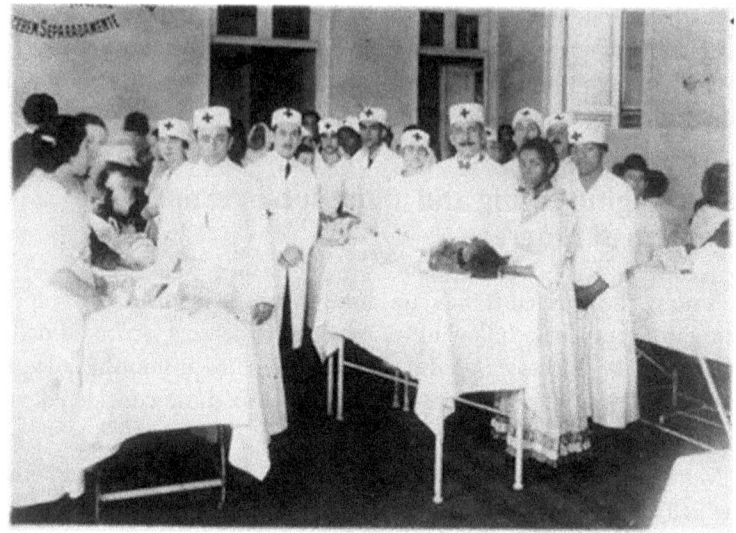

Figure 5. Os médicos Moncorvo Filho e Orlando de Góes atendendo pacientes no surto de gripe espanhola de 1918.

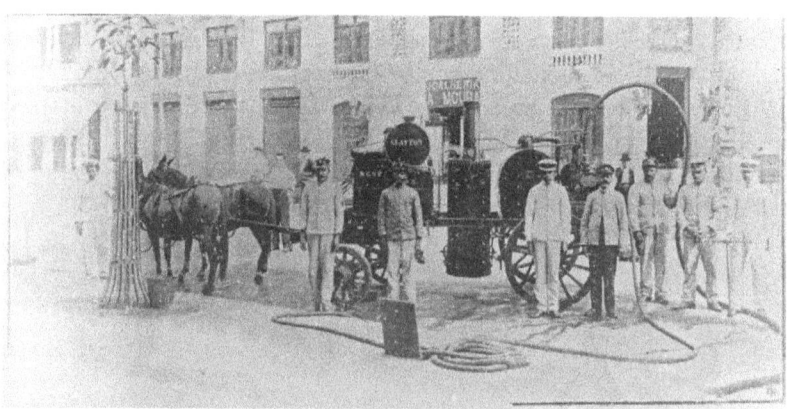

Figure 6. Clayton devices for terrestrial prophylaxis services.

The picture of the Yellow Fever Prophylaxis Service, in turn, presents us not with sick bodies but with a team staged before a lens: the team prepares for a disinfection process using the Clayton Apparatus – a machine invented in 1903 which emits a dry sulfurous gas compound effective for decontaminating objects and against disease-carrying animals, such as rats and bedbugs.

These images were taken in the early 20th century, a time of effervescence of the sanitary movement in Brazil, especially due to the campaigns of the 1910s and 1920s. It also saw the consolidation of health as a state-managed collective good and a manifest belief in the normalizing power of the hygiene sciences, as mentioned. Hence, beyond what is seen in the images – frames depicting the bodies qualified to combat pathological agents – we note a historical framing according to which science would be the one responsible for overcoming Brazil's "backwardness".

At the same time, the power of the medical dispositif and the Brazilian sanitary movement was followed by the consolidation of a certain identity imputed to part of the Brazilian population – the sick. Such an identity is highlighted in the famous speech by Miguel Pereira (1871–1918),[5] delivered in October 1916, from which derives the maxim "O Brasil é ainda um imenso hospital" [Brazil remains one huge hospital]:

> Outside Rio or São Paulo, more or less sanitized capitals, and some or other cities where welfare oversees hygiene, *Brazil remains one huge hospital*. In an impressive display of oratory, the illustrious parliamentarian has already stated that, if it were necessary, he would go from mountain to mountain, awakening the caboclos of these backlands. Such an extreme example of patriotic zeal, his generous and noble initiative would be received with great disappointment. A considerable part of this brave people would not rise; crippled, drained, exhausted by hookworm disease and malaria; maimed and ravaged by Chagas disease; corroded by syphilis and leprosy; devastated by alcoholism; sucked dry by hunger, ignorant, abandoned, without an ideal and illiterate, or could these sad forgotten people rise from their slumber to the shrill call of a warrior trumpet, [...] or when, like specters, they would rise, they would not be able to understand why the Homeland, which denied them the alphabet, now asks them for life and in their hands, before the redeeming book, put the defensive weapon. (PEREIRA, 1922 [1916]: 6)

---

[5] Miguel da Silva Pereira was a sanitary doctor, professor, and member of the National Academy of Medicine.

The speech was delivered at the reception to Aloysio de Castro, then director of the Faculty of Medicine of Rio de Janeiro who had returned from Argentina and took place amidst debates about conscription and compulsory military service. Pereira was referring especially to the declarations of Congressman Carlos Peixoto, when he proclaimed that, in face of the world conflict taking place, he would be willing to summon the countryside population to join the Brazilian army and defend the country (Sá, 2009). Pereira mocks the Congressperson's speech by inferring that this population was predominantly sick due to the continued abandonment by the public power. The statement is considered a turning point in the face of interpretations about the "Brazilian disease" commonly based on geographical and biological determinism. Pereira's statement, thus, was a milestone for attributing the poor health conditions to the absence of state management.

This speech also results from Pereira's reading of a report published by physicians Artur Neiva and Belisário Penna on the health, hygiene and salubrious life conditions of the countryside populations, after a seven-month research in several regions of Brazil. The diagnosis detailed issues such as the climate, the fauna, the flora and the diseases that affected the inhabitants of those regions. It also pointed not only to their lack of identification with the Brazilian nation project but also to the omnipresence of endemics, the result of precarious living conditions. The study called for prophylactic actions to prevent the spread of these evils and argued that this "rediscovered" Brazil was a Brazil whose population had been forgotten and abandoned.

Thus, Miguel Pereira was aware that recognizing Brazil as a territory of sick populations meant that instead of resigned attitude, one could overcome a precarious condition through hygiene, sanitation and policies aimed at improving the health of those peoples (Lima & Hochman, 2000). However, such perception brings forth framings that assign specific places to specific subjects. In other words, these framings enclose bodies in lives subject to suffering, vulnerable bodies and combat-qualified bodies – a discursive construction of life that draws on the semantics of war and the moral judgement that defines who is fit or unfit to live and make live.

Thinking a possible constellation in which caring and ailing bodies escape the staged portrait

Despite the predominance of biopolitical framings in the images, we noted a potency of figuration, especially when the medical team tried to recreate conditions of contact, either between physicians and patients, or between patients and their families. Certain images hint at an agency that produces gaps and intervals in consensual semantics, bringing, according to Didi-Huberman (2017 [2009]) and Rancière (2021), other mechanisms of legibility of history, the ordinary and experience, differing from the explanatory framings of representation that add symbolic violence to already oppressed subjects.

To make suffering subjects appear, we must consider them as alive and powerful, always moving, doing their tasks and being able to change their conditions of vulnerability. Hence, the act examining people on the street on a rainy day while at work, performed by some physicians during the Spanish flu, place the sick back into their contexts of experience, valuing their efforts to preserve their lifestyle, their mobility and their agency.

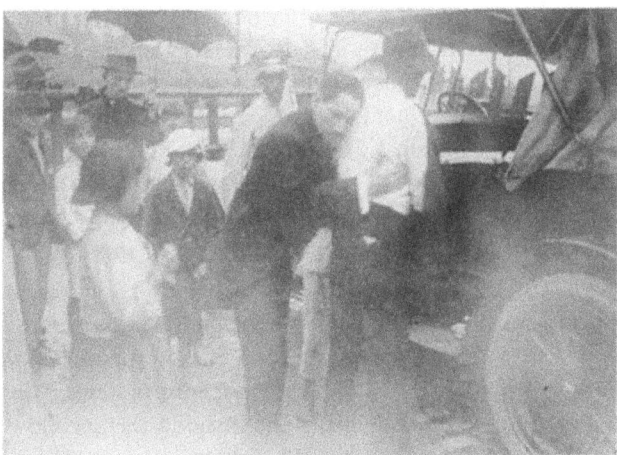

Figure 7. Doctor Peregrino Silva examining people on Morro da Mangueira during the Spanish flu epidemic of 1918. Dr. Peregrino da Silva; examining a grippe-affected adult; at Mangueira Station; on a rainy day.

Elaborating a way of life is to think about a relational process that ensures life-sustaining networks. It involves considering that the world in which we act and perform moral acts is a material, affective and institutional arrangement that conditions our acts and possibilities of life. Thus, what makes us act comes from social and moral formations articulated, implicitly or explicitly, in an extremely material reality (FASSIN, 2016 [2015]).

For Ferrarese and Laugier (2018: 12), a way of life always entails a succession of practices or even a maintenance work, of continuous engendering and production that draws on learnings derived from life as a "form created while living". It is about acting in unscripted ways, articulating the knowledge of experience to put into practice resources that ensure survival conditions. Thus, to elaborate a way of life is to engage in a patient work of ethical orientation regarding oneself and others. For these authors, the ethical texture of life has a logic of articulation, describing the slow aggregation of meaning-laden practices that are, in the course of this process, progressively transformed into the material that alters the course of experiences of vulnerability.

One clear way to detect a way of living, according to Marielle Macé (2018 [2017]), is the loss of the routine structure that is performed everyday (in situations of extreme precariousness, disasters, migrations, epidemics, and collective traumas), because the dismantling of the habitual network that ensures existences connects the vulnerability of social forms and norms to a radical vulnerability of ways of life and of living. These situations of fracture and loss of social and material life-sustaining networks imply the slow work of redefining how life counts as important and which spaces of freedom, happiness, inventiveness and change can be realized, elaborated and unfolded from moments of rupture.

Fassin (2016 [2015]) argues that the concept of ways of life allows us not to underestimate how people reinvent their trajectories, giving special emphasis to the potentialities they endow themselves with, the resources they mobilize, the tactics they put into practice, the achievements they attain, and the solidarities and imaginaries that allow them to escape, at least in part, the constraints weighing on them. Although their actions are constantly limited by precariousness, the image above shows how people deploy tactical resources to deal with institutional, social and health constraints, while public authorities fret before the powerful affections, "gambiarras" and bricolages they cannot master.

In images showing the tactics employed by ICU staff responsible treating Covid-19 patients, we see how the use of electronic devices such as tablets and cell phones could reconnect patients with their families, challenging the predictability of consensual rationality and creating an experimental and dissenting narrative (Rancière, 2021). The medical team was able to fracture protocols based on a different way of thinking and performing a distribution and organization of bodies, circumventing social isolation and questioning the positions and rules already pointed out. This gesture of connection created gaps in the controlled conditions of visibility, consideration, listening and recognition of the subjects. What we see in the images below is the creation of a political potency of consideration which, according to Macé (2018 [2017]), involves apprehending ways of life as procedural rather than as frozen moments based on essentializing and dehumanizing frames. Hence, for Butler (2015 [2009]), vulnerability is not immutable but can be modified as the individual alters the conditions of his experience, experiencing forms of individual and collective agency.

The documentary also goes back to the fact that if there are biopolitical frames that focus on bodies, let us take up the Foucauldian argument that life as a political object was taken and, somehow, turned against the system that intended to control it (Foucault, 1981 [1979]). Some interpreters, in elaborating an exegesis of Foucault's thought, argue that this power over life is sometimes interpellated by a power of life – by some called biopotency (Pelbart, 2016 [2003]). This power of life consists in what makes its forms vary and reinvents its coordinates of enunciation. Biopotency lets us glimpse the fact that life forms do not constitute an "inert and passive mass [...], but a set of strategies" (Pelbart, 2016 [2003]: 21), from which new meanings, becoming, and devices of valorization and self-valorization are created. Put another way, biopower can act on power over life, since it reveals situated vulnerabilities and acts in defining what counts as life, without underestimating the potentialities, tactics, achievements, imaginaries and solidarities that allow them to escape the constraints that weigh upon them. With this in view, we argue that it is not up to biopolitics inadvertently to produce bare life, a life devoid of form.

We can think, in this way, these images as dispositifs that transform power over life into the potency of life. About the constraints and coercions of the biopolitical apparatus, Valérie Marange (2000) calls attention to the literary accounts of survivors of concentration camps during the Second World War. According to the author, such testimonies point to a dimension of vital affirmation, in opposition to the politics of extermination – so that the very idea of bare life implies a reduction of life, in the face of its multiple capacities for action in the operations of power.

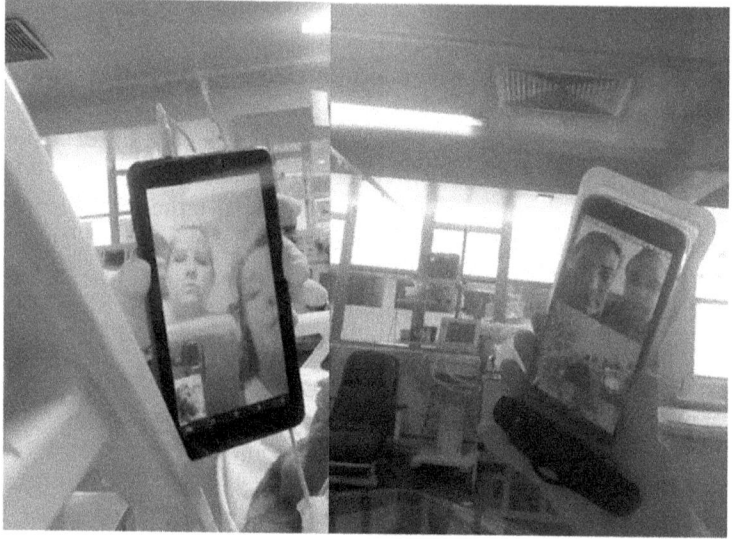

Figures 8 and 9. Frames of "Estamos te esperando em casa".

These images from Cecília da Fonte and Marcelo Pedroso's documentary film reveal intervals or gaps in which intelligibility about the event/the other escapes any clear and closed understanding, provoking tensions and contradictions (Rancière, 2018). Thus, this tactic of consideration emerges as a possibility to dismantle a hegemonic visibility and temporality, which standardize subjects and their experiences, neglecting their complexities, intersectionalities, support networks and capabilities as multifaceted and dignified individuals, able to traverse through conditions and places of vulnerability.

Macé (2018 [2017]) also states that consideration entails a movement of surprise towards the life and experience of others, beyond their contact with pain and vulnerability. In other words, it is about listening to what the other enunciates not from suffering, but in spite of it. Those who survive have hopes, dreams, ideals, habits, passions and preferences that cross their existence and make up their agency in everyday life. "To consider would be to take into account the living, their actual lives, since it is in this way and in no other that these lives are stolen from the present—to take into account their practices, their days, and then liberate what sideration encloses; not to assign and label victims, but to describe everything each one puts into action to deal with situations of vulnerability" (Macé, 2018 [2017]: 28).

The images from "Estamos te esperando em casa" show care as a political tool of resistance, inventiveness and desires for strengthening affections, exposing doubts and producing alternatives capable of feeding dreams and becoming. These minor experiences reveal how the image also works to promote openings for unforeseen connections, shuffling the relationships between those who produce the images (medical and nursing staff), the figured subject (patients), and the spectators (family members). The contract is not to look at pain or simply sympathize but to lift up the suffering faces – to open gaps for the potent affection of love, friendship and hospitality. If, on the one hand, the pedagogies of cruelty, according to Rita Segato (2021), allow the repetition of violence which normalizes cruelty, the pedagogy of love, by bell hooks (2021), engenders a transformative culture that breaks with an ethics of domination and continued allegiance to systems of domination (imperialism, sexism, racism, classism). Love and friendship fracture the pedagogy of cruelty, the acts and practices capable of habituating and programming subjects to reify what is alive. The pedagogy of cruelty feeds an action that does not recognize the other as a being, excluding and condemning them.

Cecília da Fonte and Marcelo Pedroso's film creates other framings to represent and read the images, which allow operations and arrangements that show the survival of ways of life, highlighting their agency and autonomy as a way of acting which produces an inhabitable world. Institutional control acts by defining what a human life is and what counts as life, underestimating the potentialities, tactics, achievements, imaginaries and solidarities that allow them to escape their constraints (Butler, 2019 [2014]). As survivors, they create a way of life that ensures them a face to be contemplated in a game of enunciation and invention of resistances.

To care is to search for a "humanity" lost in the exhausting work of remaking everyday life: those who make and maintain a way of life must also be cared for and care for others around them, nurturing an ethical relationship of responsibility and continuous attention that preserves dignity and life. According to Ferrarese and Laugier (2018), caring requires a sensitivity to the details that count in lived situations, since they need preservation and constant repair of all dimensions, links and articulations that, precisely because they are not negligible, require great physical, moral and ethical work.

Images can thus be operators of dissensus and make the unexpected appear, that which was previously unperceived, perceived, felt: they produce and are produced by operations that disorganize, disturb and rearrange what is given, defining other possibilities, that is, other ways of making times, spaces, objects, bodies, and experiences legible and intelligible. Images can give rise to singular and fabulous scenes by playing the role of "small machines that refuse the explanation already given" (Rancière, 2019: 57).

Bibliography

Butler, Judith (2009). *Quadros de Guerra*. Quando a vida é passível de luto? Rio de Janeiro: Civilização Brasileira, 2015.

Butler, Judith (2012). *Caminhos Divergentes*. São Paulo: Boitempo, 2017.

Butler, Judith (2014). *Vida precária*. Belo Horizonte: Autêntica, 2019.

Castro-Santos, Luiz (1985). "O pensamento sanitarista na Primeira República: Uma ideologia de construção de nacionalidade". *Dados - Revista de Ciências Sociais*, 28 (2), 193–210.

Chalhoub, Sidney (1996). *Cidade febril: Cortiços e epidemias na corte imperial*. São Paulo: Companhia das Letras, 2018.

Didi-Huberman, Georges (2011). *Atlas Ou Le Gai Savoir Inquiet*. L'Oeil De L'Histoire. 3. Paris : Éditions de Minuit.

Didi-Huberman, Georges (2004). *Images in Spite of All: Four Photographs from Auschwitz* (1st ed.). Illinois: University of Chicago Press, 2012.

Didi-Huberman, Georges (2013). "Povos expostos, povos figurantes". *Vista: Revista de Cultura Visual*, 1 (1), 16–31. https://doi.org/10.1590/S1517-106X2013000200014, 2017.

Didi-Huberman, Georges (2009). *Quando as Imagens Tomam Posição: o Olho da História, I*. Belo Horizonte: Editora UFMG, 2019.

De Cauwer, Stijn (2018). Searching for fireflies: Pathos and imagination in the theories of Georges didi-huberman. Angelaki 23 (4):133-149.

Fassin, Didier (2015). "The Value of Life and the Worth of Lives", in *Living and Dying in the Contemporary World*: A Compendium, DAS, Veena and HAN, Clara (eds.). California: The Regents of the University of California, Library of Congress, 770–783, 2016.

Ferrarese, Estelle and Laugier, Sandra (2018). *Formes de vie*. Paris: CNRS Éditions.

Foucault, Michel (1979). *Microfísica do poder*. Rio de Janeiro: Edições Graal Ltda, 1981.

Freire, Maria Martha and Leony, Vinicius (2011). "A caridade científica: Moncorvo Filho e o Instituto de Proteção e Assistência à Infância do Rio de Janeiro (1899–1930)". *História, Ciências, Saúde-Manguinhos*, 18, 199–225. https://doi.org/10.1590/S0104-59702011000500011

Goulart, Adriana da Costa (2005), « Revisitando a espanhola: a gripe pandêmica de 1918 no Rio de Janeiro ». *História, Ciências, Saúde – Manguinhos*, v. 12, n. 1, pp. 101-42.

Hochman, Gilberto. (1998). *A era do saneamento: As bases da política de saúde pública no Brasil*. São Paulo: Editora Hucitec, 2011.

hooks, bell (2021). "O amor como ato de liberdade". *Anânsi: Revista de Filosofia*, Salvador, v. 2, n. 2, 277–283.

Lima, Nísia and Hochman, Gilberto (2000). "Pouca saúde, muita saúva, os males do Brasil são... Discurso médico-sanitário e interpretação do país", *Ciência & Saúde Coletiva*, 5, 313–332. https://doi.org/10.1590/S1413-81232000000200007

Macé, Marielle (2017). *Siderar, considerar: migrantes, formas de vida*. Rio de Janeiro: Bazar do Tempo, 2018.

Machado, Roberto (1978). *Danação da norma: Medicina social e constituição da psiquiatria no* Brasil: Graal.

Marange, Valérie (2000). L'inavouable, politique, perception et folie. **Chimères. Revue des schizoanalyses**, v. 39, n. 1, 53–62.

Mitchell, William John Thomas (2016). "Method, Madness and Montage: Assemblages of Images and the Production of Knowledge", in *Image Operations*, Eden and Klonk (eds.), Visual Media and Manchester, 79–85. Manchester: Manchester University Press.

Müller, Maristela (2018). "Conhecimento por Montagem: Aproximações e Diferenças em Didi-Huberman, Warburg e Eisenstein", *Revista da Fundarte*, 35 (35), 12–29.

Pelbart, Peter Pál (2003). *Vida capital: ensaios de biopolítica*. Rio de Janeiro Editora Iluminuras Ltda, 2016.

Pereira, Miguel (1922 [1916]). "O Brasil é ainda um imenso hospital — discurso pronunciado pelo prof. Miguel Pereira por ocasião do regresso do prof. Aloysio de Castro, da República Argentina, em outubro de 1916", *Revista de Medicina — órgão do Centro Acadêmico Oswaldo Cruz/Faculdade de Medicina e Cirurgia de São Paulo*, VII (21) 3–7.

Rancière, Jacques (2017). *Les bords de la fiction*. Paris: Éditions du Seuil.

Rancière, Jacques (2018). *Le temps modernes*. Paris: La Fabrique.

Rancière, Jacques (2019). *Le travail des images. Conversations avec Andrea Soto Calderón*. Dijon: Les Presses du Réel.

Rancière, Jacques (2021). O método da cena. Belo Horizonte: Quixote+DO.

Rego, José Pereira (1851). *História de descrição da febre amarela epidêmica que grassou no Rio de Janeiro em 1850*. Belo Horizonte: Chão Editora, 2020.

Sá, Dominichi Miranda (2009). "A voz do Brasil: Miguel Pereira e o discurso sobre o imenso hospital". *História, Ciências, Saúde-Manguinhos*, 16, 333–348. https://doi.org/10.1590/S0104-59702009000500016

Santos, Boaventura de Sousa (2021). *O futuro começa agora: Da pandemia à utopia*. São Paulo: Boitempo.

Schwarcz, Lília Moritz and Starling Heloísa (2020). *A bailarina da morte: A gripe espanhola no* Brasil: Companhia das Letras.

Schwarte, Ludger (2018). "The People Image", *Angelaki*, 23 (4), 80–90, DOI: 10.1080/0969725X.2018.1497281

Segato, Rita Laura (2021). *Contra-pedagogías de la crueldad*. Buenos Aires: Prometeo.

Silveira, Anny Jackeline Torres. (2008). *A influenza espanhola e a cidade planejada: Belo Horizonte, 1918*. Belo Horizonte: Fino Traço.

Weizman, Eyal (2014). "Forensis: Introduction", in *Forensis: The Architecture of Public Truth*, Forensic Architecture (ed.), Berlin: Sternberg Press, 9–32.

Filmography

Estamos te esperando em casa, dir. Cecília da Fonte e Marcelo Pedroso, 2021.

Strategic communication and the vaccination plan of Covid-19: The Uruguayan case

PATRICIA SCHROEDER, *Universidad de Montevideo*

Introduction

This chapter is an advancement of the investigation project related to the study of the Uruguayan case. In previous works, aspects of government communication (Schroeder & Amadeo, 2021) and recently specific elements associated with the digital communication of the vaccination against Covid-19 were developed.

The Uruguayan government's management of the pandemic has been recognized as successful on a national and international level. The population has manifested their approval in public opinion polls, and President Lacalle Pou´s upstanding management is recognized globally (Uruguay XXI, 2021).

In this campaign for the mitigation of the pandemic [1], government communication and the intervention of other actors in society have played a fundamental role. From the government communication, a transmedia strategy was promoted, combining all communication platforms and intensive use of social media. These aspects were central for all areas of government and especially for the Ministry of Public Health in the implementation of a health strategy (Schroeder & Amadeo, 2021).

In a global context of high demand for vaccines against Covid-19 and a scenario of uncertainty, Uruguay has managed to position itself in the first place in the world in the advancement of vaccination. By June 2022, 84,6 % of the population had the complete vaccination schedule (Ministerio de Salud Pública– Uruguay 2021 f).

The rapid advance of the vaccination was reflected in the contention of the adverse effects of the new variants of Covid-19. The entry of the Delta Variant did not have as a consequence a significant increase in the cases, and the subsequent entry of the Omicron Variant did not have an impact on the occupation level of the ICU beds, nor on the mortality. These aspects will be analyzed later based on the analysis of the data offered by the epidemiological surveillance department of the Ministry of Public Health.

This chapter will present the communication strategy of the Covid-19 vaccination campaign developed in Uruguay until May 2022. Although at the time of writing the campaign has not been completed, it is possible to analyze its design and implementation. The theoretical frame that supports the strategy will be explained, combining concepts of strategic communication with others of government communication, health communication, and risk communication.

Government communication is held with digital communication support, offline media and communication of authorities in the territory. Digital communication channels and new technologies have played a fundamental role due to the need to carry out an unprecedented campaign in terms of the logistics required and the target audience to be reached. Digital communication allowed, among other relevant aspects, to keep the public opinion informed in real-time about the available agenda (day and time of vaccination according to their group), vaccination progress (vaccine monitor), vaccines available in the country, and reports on safety and efficacy of vaccines.

To explain the communication strategy of the Covid-19 vaccination, it is useful to make a brief reference to the social-political aspects of Uruguay. It should be noted that the campaign started in a climate of uncertainty. Afterward, a resume of the theoretical framework was exposed, and finally, a description of the distinctive aspects of the communication strategy of the Covid-19 vaccination campaign in Uruguay was offered.

Research methodology

As it was mentioned before, this study is an extension and actualization of the information concerning the contributions of digital communication collected in Schroeder, 2022. The focus will be given to the communication strategy of the vaccination against Covid-19 that is close to completion.

A qualitative study was conducted during the period February 2021–May 2022. First, the initial context of uncertainty is described, followed by a brief mention of the epidemiological situation – a list of the main communication challenges – and then an analysis of the development of the message in several formats.

As already mentioned, digital communication had a preponderant place because it allowed reaching a large audience. It also enabled the segmentation of messages and contents according to specific audiences.

The pieces analyzed are those available to public opinion in the official networks of the Ministry of Public Health. Likewise, the reports of the work meetings of the communication team that participated in the communication strategy of the Ministry of Public Health were studied.

A quantitative study of the followers in the social networks of the Ministry of Public Health and their evolution was carried out. Additionally, a survey of official content published on social networks and website news was also included.

Concerning the analysis of the media, the information was monitored in the morning and evening central news programs on Channel 4, Channel 12, Channel 10, and Channel 5; as well as the following in written press: the newspapers *El País*, *El Observador*, and *La República*, plus the weekly newspapers *Search* and *Brecha*.

Finally, the content of the ministry's social networks and also the Twitter and Instagram of both, Minister Salinas and Undersecretary Satdjian, were also included in this analysis.

Theoretical framework

Before proceeding with the description of the vaccination communication strategy, it is pertinent to briefly develop the theoretical framework that supports it. The contributions of the conceptual framework developed by Schroeder (2022) are used.

Different theories have been applied in health communication campaigns. Among the most frequent are, on the one hand, social science theories that explain what drives people's behavior and how these can be modified; on the other hand, communication theories in which what stands out is that the source, the channel, the receiver, and the message are essential components. In these two groups of theories, it is concluded that information does not fall into a social vacuum but is received through processes of exposure and selective perception, prior knowledge, and macro-social levels (Tench & Bridge 2021).

Authors Tench and Bridge highlight three theories or models: the Theory of Planned Behavior, the Likelihood Model, and the Extended Parallel Process Model.

The Theory of Planned Behavior (Ajzen, 1985) proposes that voluntary action is a function of the individual's intention to perform a behavior and perceived control. Therefore, for a successful health communication campaign, the message must consider the target audience's attitudes about the behavior, their subjective norms, and levels of perceived behavioral control.

The Likelihood Model (Cacioppo & Petty, 1984; Petty & Cacioppo, 1986) has been applied to improve health outcomes for several health problems, including smoking, nutrition, and reduction of risk behaviors concerning acquired immunodeficiency syndrome (AIDS). It focuses on asking how people will react to the messages to which they will be exposed.

The Extended Parallel Process Model, based on the health belief model (Rosenstock et al., 1992), analyzes the role of emotions in behavior change. Studies on the topic show that while fear is a factor that positively influences a behavior change, it can become detrimental if people become paralyzed (Tench R. & Bridge. G., 2021). The authors conclude that fear should be used with caution in health campaigns, and the sensitivity of the target audience and their ability to make changes should be taken into account.

Authors Tench and Bridge (2021) conclude that all three models emphasize that for health communication campaigns to be successful, the communication strategy must consider the target audience, their subjective norms, and perceptions of health behavior. Also, messages should be clear and understandable to the target audience. It is necessary to evaluate whether the audience is engaged in the message or it is needed to find a way to capture their attention. And, in the case of using fear to change behavior, the relationship between fear and motivation to change should be measured because fear can lead to paralysis.

Finally, it is worth mentioning Schiavo's contributions. (Schiavo, R., 2013, 32–46) explains the different theoretical approaches that influence the development of public health campaigns. Families of social and behavioral science theories, mass communication and social marketing theories, and other models that include medical, sociological, and anthropological models are highlighted.

The following theories and models were selected because they are useful to understand the vaccination communication strategy.

The Innovation Theory (Rogers & Kinkaid, 1981; Rogers 1995) addresses how new ideas, concepts, or practices can be spread within a community and defines five subgroups: innovators, early adopters, early majority, late majority, and laggards. The fundamental premise is that change occurs over time and depends on the following stages: awareness, knowledge and interest, decision, testing and implementation, confirmation, and rejection.

The Health Belief Model (Becker, Haefner, & Maiman, 1977; Janz & Becker, 1984; Strecher & Rosenstock, 1997) explains that to adopt healthy patterns, individuals must be aware of the risks of serious or life-threatening illnesses. They must also perceive the benefits of behavior change. The fundamental premise of this theory is that knowledge will bring about behavior change.

The Social Cognitive Theory (Bandura, 1997) explains behavior as a result of three reciprocal factors: behavior, personal factors, and external events. One of the fundamental premises is its emphasis on the external factors, and its major contribution to health communications is to understand the mechanisms and factors that can influence retention, reproduction, and motivation on behavior.

The Convergence Theory (Kincaid, 1979; Rogers & Kincaid, 1981; Figueroa, Kincaid, Rani & Lewis, 2002) is based on the perspective that an individual's perceptions and behavior are influenced by the perceptions and behaviors of members of the same group, such as professional associations, coworkers, family members, and people in one's social media.

Finally, the Communication for Persuasion Theory developed by social psychologist William Mc Guire focuses on how people process information. According to this model, in the process of persuasive communication, there are twelve steps. For a person to change their behavior they must be exposed to the message, pay attention, find it interesting or personally relevant, understand it, find out how this new behavior can fit into their life, accept the proposed change, remember and validate the message, be able to think about the message in relevant situations, make decisions based on the information, behave according to that decision, receive positive reinforcement for that behavior, and integrate the new behavior into their life (Moya, 2000).

We must add health communication models designed for risk communication and evidence-based communication to these existing conceptual frameworks (Tormo, M. J., Banegas, J. R. 2001; Nespereira, J. 2014; Schwarzinger, M., & Luchini, S. 2021). It is also supported by the government communication implemented to date in the context of Covid-19 (Schroeder & Amadeo, 2021).

Risk communication frames should help to avoid contradictions to reinforce the credibility of government communication (González-Melado, F. J., & Di Pietro, M. L. 2020; Rzymski, P., Borkowski, L., Drąg, M., Flisiak, R., Jemielity, J., Krajewski, J., Mastalerz-Migas, A., et al. 2021).

Risk communication also requires permanent monitoring of the epidemiological situation to know the evolution of the pandemic and the reactions of the population. Specifically, in the Uruguayan case, the beginning of vaccination coincided with an increment in the number of cases. This factor required, on the one hand, reinforcing the concept that vaccines are effective in minimizing the pandemic, which would bring about a decrease in contagion and consequently a decrease in the number of deaths. On the other hand, the increment in cases elevates the perception of risk and was a factor that most likely contributed favorably to accelerating vaccination.

From the perspective of risk communication, the following issues collaborate in a successful communication (Moreno & Peres, 2020).

The source responsible for the transmission of information must have credibility –

(1) honesty. What is not known must be reported and clarified.
(2) Meaningful actions that help to understand the message.
(3) Participation of experts regarding medical issues and in risk communication.
(4) Consistency in messages.

In the next chapter, data about the social, political, and health situation of the country will be offered, with the purpose of achieving a better understanding of the development of communication in traditional social media and the territory.

Uruguay´s characteristics: *Government system, population and health system*

In the following lines, aspects related to Uruguay´s political situation, the government system, the geographical location, the density of the population, and the political climate before the arrival of the vaccine will be developed in order to achieve a better understanding of the communication strategy during the pandemic and specifically the implementation of an unprecedented vaccination in the country's history.

Government system

The Uruguayan case and aspects related to the communication of the pandemic were narrated by Schroeder & Amadeo (2021). The authors explain in the Introduction that the Uruguayan government system is a representative presidential democracy and that it combines forms of direct government such as the referendum and the plebiscite. It has three powers: Executive (made up of the president and his council of ministers), a bicameral Legislative Power, and a Judicial Power headed by the Supreme Court of Justice.

The president, vice president, and the members of both chambers are elected for five years on the same date. The 19 municipal governments are elected two months after the president takes office, and they become part of a centralized administration.

In November 2019, the Lacalle Pou-Argimón formula won with the support of an electoral coalition composed of five parties: *Partido Nacional, Partido Colorado, Cabildo Abierto, Partido Independiente,* and *Partido De La Gente.*

As part of this electoral agreement, some ministries were occupied by politicians and technicians from different areas of the coalition: specifically, the Minister of Public Health, Dr. Daniel Salinas, is a neurologist and trusted person of the leader of Cabildo Abierto, and Lic. José Luis Satdjian, the undersecretary of that ministry, leads one of the young political forces of the Partido Nacional (Schroeder & Amadeo, 2021).

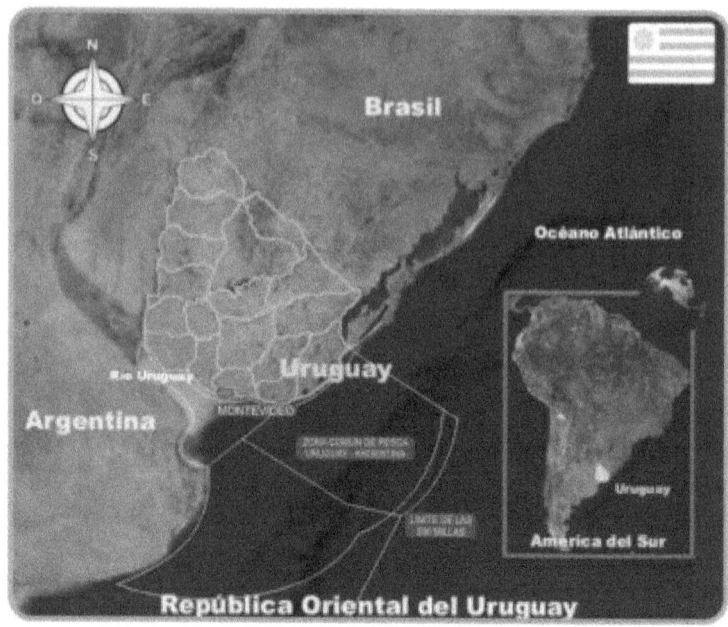

Figure 1. National territory (National Institute of Statistics in Schroeder and Amadeo, 2021).

Geographic location and population density

The authors also give data about the geographic location and demography of the country.

They highlight that the country occupies a total land area of 176,215 km^2. It has a border with Brazil, Argentina, and the Atlantic Ocean (Figure 1).

Concerning the number of inhabitants, the 2011 national census indicated that Uruguay has 3,286,314 inhabitants. It has a high degree of urbanization (92.8 %), and 40 % of the population is concentrated in Montevideo (the capital city) and two other departments: Canelones and Maldonado (Figure 2).

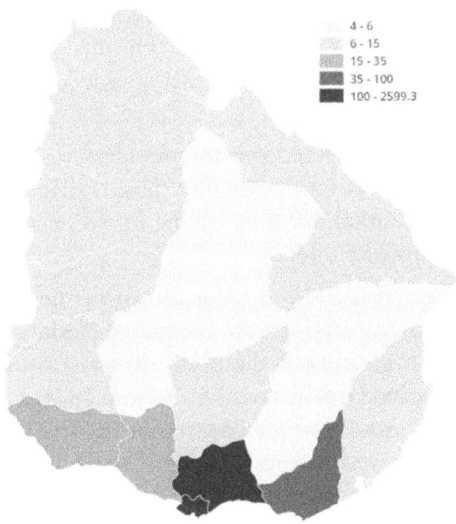

Figure 2. Population (per 100,000 inhabitants) (National Institute of Statistics and Census in Schroeder and Amadeo, 2021).

Health system

According to Oreggiani (2015), Uruguay begins the gestation process of the current health system early. Mutual organizations were first created in the first half of the 19th century. The first mutual organizations emerged, currently called Collective Medical Assistance Institutions (IAMC). These institutions were financed from the beginning with a system based on the principles of solidarity and mutual aid. Initially, they brought together groups of people who shared some aspects in common (e.g., the Spanish Association of Mutual Aid or Casa de Galicia, brought together descendants of immigrants). They quickly grew in the number of affiliates, and this feature that summoned affiliates was lost over the years.

This coverage was not enough to provide universal assistance due to the diverse economic possibilities of the different sectors of the population. At the beginning of 1900, the government began to offer medical assistance to the most deprived sectors, and this process reached a milestone in 1933 with the creation of the Ministry of Public Health with an assistance role rather than a stewardship role.

Over time, different public providers were formed, such as ASSE (the largest health provider in the country), the Hospital Militar, the Hospital Policial, and the municipal polyclinics that are added to the already existing mutual insurance companies.

In this system of public and private providers, universal assistance is provided, but differences in accessibility persist, determined mainly by the ability to pay a mutual fee or by paying for services (through tickets) that each private provider offers.

To develop the articulation of the actors of the health system and to ensure the quality of the services, the Integrated National Health System was created at the beginning of the 21st century (Law 18,211 of 5/12/2007 and later modified by the laws 18,731 and 18,732 of 7/1/2011). It is worth bearing in mind that the creation of the INHS allowed greater integration of public and private providers and a financing model for health care. As a consequence, all workers in the public and private sectors must contribute a percentage of their salary (this percentage varies depending on whether or not they have dependent children).

It should be noted that the INHS constituted a strength in the management of the pandemic because it allowed the development of health strategies during the first phase in the monitoring of cases and outbreaks. When the cases increased and the health system was stressed, national coordination of ICU beds was implemented, which resulted in the system not collapsing despite the saturation in some areas of the country.

Uruguay was also a pioneer in the development of emergency medical care at home at the end of the last century. The Mobile Coronary Unit was the first company in Latin America to develop this home ambulance service. Others followed, such as SEMM and SUAT, among others. This home care was also a strength during the first year of the pandemic since it allowed the care of patients without them going to hospital centers.

Telemedicine was also improved, and thus a greater follow-up of patients was achieved by telephone or with the WhatsApp application.

After this brief analysis of the political, social and demographic conditions of Uruguay, some aspects that were decisive in the communication strategy are concluded:

(1) The Uruguayan government faced a great challenge with a coalition government of five parties, and this led to a consensus communication with a parliamentary majority.

(2) The presidential political system facilitated coordinated action throughout the national territory.

(3) The land borders with Brazil were a critical point in combating the pandemic.

(4) The population concentrated in the capital and the cities throughout the territory allowed, on the one hand, rapid progress in vaccination. On the other hand, it implied a challenge to reach remote places in the country.

These aspects illustrate the double role of communication: to achieve very high levels of trust in governmental decisions and to achieve a general behavior that accompanies this vaccination process.

In the next chapter a general description of the political and epidemiological climate will be described, because it´s useful to understand the government communication developed.

Political climate before vaccination: Uncertainty

The climate of uncertainty and its communicational challenges were presented by Schroeder (2022). The communication of all aspects related to Covid-19 has uncertainty as a common denominator. As never before, scientific knowledge has been within the reach of governments and public opinion. However, political decisions to confront a pandemic of these dimensions must be executed quickly, and the production of scientific knowledge has its deadlines, not always according to political times.

Uncertainty is compounded by *Infodemic* that brings with it excessive amounts of information and misinformation (Schroeder & Amadeo, 2021). In a vaccination campaign, trust in vaccines as the main measure to mitigate harm is essential. Just as communication plays a fundamental role in getting people to adopt personal protection measures (physical distance, use of masks, and hand washing, in addition to social behaviors that lead to not crowding), in this phase of the pandemic 70 % of the population must agree to be vaccinated (according to scientific recommendations at that moment).

Although in the first year of the pandemic, the opposition party had a moderated attitude, as the pandemic worsened due to the appearance of new, more aggressive strains, the opposition exerted greater pressure for the start of vaccination.

Epidemiological situation before vaccination

According to Schroeder (2022), Uruguay went through the first eight months of the pandemic without suffering the globally known as the first or second wave. The behavior of the virus during the first nine months was by outbreaks and with almost complete social mobility. The most affected sectors of the economy were tourism and those related to festivals and parties. There was an almost total closure of borders and suspension of social activities involving more than 100 people. The rest of the economic, social, educational, and sporting activities were maintained with adjustments according to the health situation.

However, in November 2020 there was an increase in cases and deaths that worsened with the presence of the P1 variant from March to June 2021 (Figure 3).

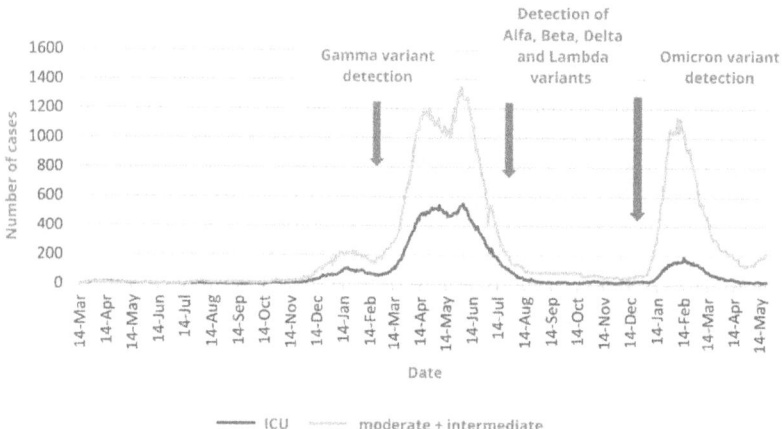

Figure 3. Number of Covid-19 confirmed cases in intensive care and intermediate care per day. From "Informe Epidemiológico", by Ministerio de Salud Pública, 2022b.

This increment in cases was the reason for more pressure from the opposition political force and also greater anxiety among the population for the arrival of the vaccine (Miranda criticó la lentitud del gobierno y dijo que es necesario tomar medidas urgentes. El presidente del Frente Amplio dijo además que el partido tiene numerosos vínculos para acelerar la llegada de la vacuna si es necesario. [Miranda criticized the government's slowness and said urgent action is needed. The president of the Frente Amplio also said that the party has numerous links to accelerate the arrival of the vaccine if necessary.], 2021; Vacunas: el FA suma presión al gobierno con nuevas críticas por falta de transparencia. [Vaccines: the FA adds pressure to the government with new criticism for lack of transparency.], 2021).

The pressure continued for several months, even after vaccination began on February 27, 2021, due to a sustained increase in cases and deaths.

In this climate of political and social tension, the authorities of the Ministry of Public Health were summoned to give explanations about the process of study and purchase of Covid-19 vaccines. On January 5, a delegation from the Ministry of Public Health and the Secretary of the Presidency attended the Senate Chamber's Health Commission (Ministerio de Salud Pública – Uruguay, 2021g).

At this commission, the Ministry of Public Health delegation explained the purchasing process managed through Covax Fund and also through bilateral negotiations. Likewise, available information was shared about the safety and efficacy of the vaccines available with Phase III studies, and the recommendations of the National Vaccine Advisory Commission and ad hoc group.

Finally, on January 23, 2021, President Lacalle Pou announced the arrival of the first vaccines. The message was received with great acceptance and partially relieved the pressure of public opinion. The government's decision was the first major purchase of vaccines from the laboratories Sinovac and Pfizer Biontech (Uruguay Presidencia, 2021a). With this first purchase, 70 % of the target population could be vaccinated (at that date the population over 18 years of age was considered, estimated at 2,836,000 people). Later, that number was expanded with the approval of vaccination for children under 18 years old.

It is worth mentioning that this purchase was made in a complex and uncertain international context, where there was a high global demand for vaccines and also the national climate of tension previously referred to. There was uncertainty as to whether the vaccines would arrive on time (first and second doses in a precise period), whether logistics could be organized according to the combination of two different platforms, whether there would be a response from the population, and whether there would be sufficient human resources (hiring a significant number of vaccinators), logistical requirements related to the cold chain, safety, and efficacy of vaccination.

Thus, in January 2020, a team led by the Ministry of Public Health (Minister Daniel Salinas and Vice Minister José Luis Satdjian) was consolidated to manage a complex process that includes the acquisition of vaccines, reception, distribution, and vaccination in the territory (Figure 4).

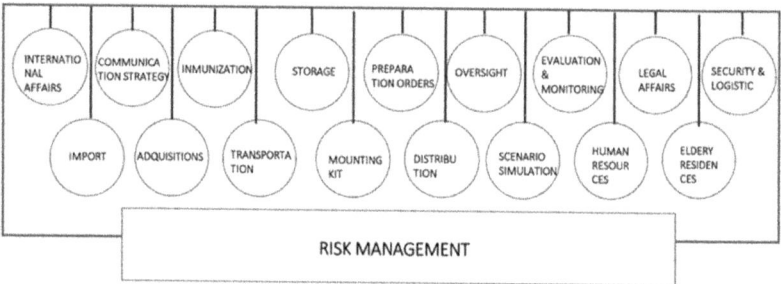

Figure 4. Integration of the team, and functional areas involved in the vaccination plan.

It is pertinent to highlight the complexity of articulating teamwork to develop a task of this magnitude in a very demanding timeframe. To this end, a vaccination plan was designed that began to be implemented on March 1 (Ministerio de Salud Pública-Uruguay 2021a), preceded by the vaccination of vaccinators on February 27 of the same year.

The first communication challenge was to establish permanent communication channels among all those involved in developing seamless communication with public opinion without contradictions.

Vaccines from the Sinovac Laboratory arrived first, and vaccination of the prioritized groups was immediately available. Then the Pfizer vaccines arrived, and all the successive arrivals were according to what was established. The vaccination plan was implemented in stages, and the main events are summarized in Figure 5.

Strategic Communication and Vaccination of Covid-19

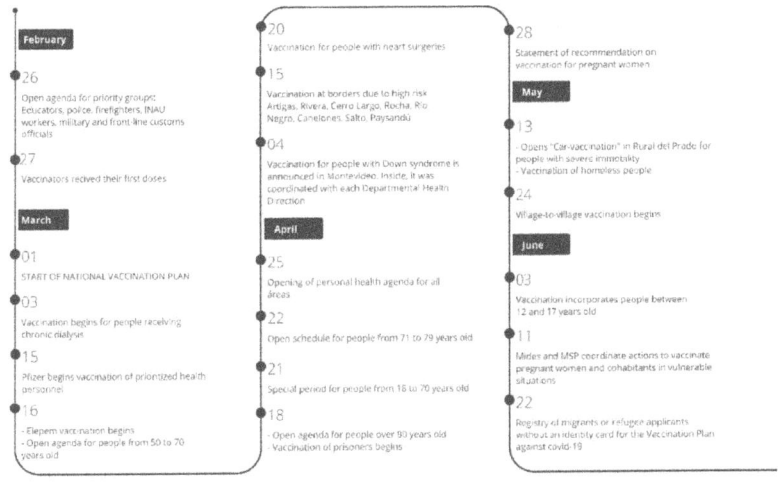

July-february

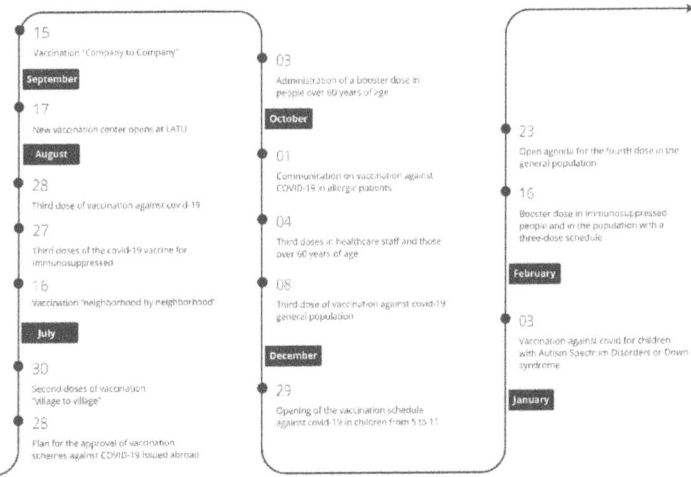

Figure 5. Main events of the vaccination plan, February 2021–February 2022.

Main challenges in designing Covid-19's communication strategy

The communication of all vaccination campaigns is challenging as it must accurately reach the previously defined target population. This is how every year since the emergence of H1N1 flu Uruguay faces the challenge of vaccinating vulnerable groups: pregnant women, children, and people over 60 years old. In 2020, in the context of the pandemic, a staggered vaccination was carried out between May and July, and the objective of vaccinating these groups was achieved. More than 950,000 doses were administered, which significantly reduced the number of respiratory infections that are typical of wintertime. This experience of staggering vaccination by groups, and with a previous schedule, served as experience to implement Covid-19 vaccination on a larger scale.

The challenges of Covid-19 vaccination are included in the recommendations of the Pan American Health Organization (Pan American Health Organization, 2021). In the Uruguayan case, the challenges are specified as follows:

1. Initially, the government set an ambitious goal: to vaccinate 70 % of the target population (over 18 years of age). With the advance of the pandemic and the analysis of the world situation, the objective became even more enthusiastic: to reach 80 % of the total population (Storlie, C. B., Pollock, B. D. Rojas, R. L., Demuth, G. O., et al 2021).

2. This is an unprecedented number; it means administering two doses of the vaccines available in the country.

3. Vaccination should be in stages. The doses would be administered to the groups defined in advance and the challenge of transmitting to the population the certainty that the plan would be executed according to the initial forecast. Vaccination began in prioritized groups, and the recommendations of the World Health Organization were used to define them.

4. Vaccines were developed in record time. The vaccines against Covid-19 were developed in a very short period, so it was necessary to transmit certainty regarding the safety and efficacy of the vaccines. In all cases, the vaccines were approved with sufficient levels of efficacy (Phase III), but in all cases – and at the time of starting vaccination in Uruguay – Phase IV studies were lacking.

5. Need for adherence in the first weeks of vaccination. For the vaccination plan to be successful, the first prioritized groups must show adherence of around 70 %. A positive first response is essential.
6. Infodemic. It is important to know how much the overabundance of information and false news about the safety and efficacy of the vaccine affects the rate of vaccination (Roozenbeek, J., Schneider, C. R., Dryhurst, S., Kerr, J., Freeman, A. L., Recchia, G., van der Bles, A. M. & van der Linden, S., 2020; Montagni, I., Ouazzani-Touhami, K., Mebarki, A., Texier, N., Schück, S., & Tzourio, C., 2021).
7. Anti-vaccine groups. It is necessary to be aware of their existence and their impact on public opinion.
8. Existence of adverse effects and how much this information may impact the vaccination campaign.
9. Maintain public confidence throughout the vaccination process, knowing in advance that there is a good chance that the plan will need to be adjusted as the epidemiological situation changes or new scientific evidence emerges.
10. Speed of vaccination. For vaccination to mitigate the pandemic, it must be carried out in an accelerated manner. This implies logistics and a territorial reach of great magnitude.

The vaccination strategy

Prior to the analysis of the communication developed for vaccination, the main aspects of the Strategic Vaccination Plan are detailed (Ministerio de Salud Pública – Uruguay, 2021b, April).

Uruguay has a National Vaccination Program (PNV) and since the 1950s it has had a commission of immunization experts called the National Vaccine Advisory Commission (CNAV), one of the oldest in America. Its main task is to provide advice to the authorities of the Ministry of Public Health regarding vaccine-preventable diseases, seeking the greatest possible vaccination coverage. It is currently made up of 15 institutions or organizations with interference in the subject. During the pandemic, they played an active role in analyzing the available vaccines for Covid-19 and their application in different age groups (Ministerio de Salud Pública n.d.).

The CNAV recommended the application of three vaccines: CoronaVac, Pfizer-BioNTech, and AstraZeneca, and the process of purchasing them was carried out by the Presidency of the Republic.

Uruguay's strategic vaccination plan frames the campaign in three principles: responsibility, solidarity, and collective good. Likewise, the campaign is following the strategic objectives defined by the WHO (World Health Organization, 2022):

Protection of the integrity of the health system and the infrastructure of essential services. In this sense, vaccination of health workers at different levels and services is recommended.

Reduction of morbidity and mortality associated with Covid-19. In this aspect, the protection of higher-risk groups is recommended.

Reduction of community infection transmission and generation of herd immunity.

The vaccination plan began with a significant amount of CoronaVac vaccine (1:742,000 doses received between February 25, 2021, and March 16, 2021) and an initial batch of 200,000 doses of the Pfizer vaccine that was received in batches of 50,000 as of March 24, 2021 (Ministerio de Salud Pública – Uruguay, 2021b, April).

In accordance with the vaccination plan, an order was made that took into account the risk of serious illness (ages and comorbidity, risk due to exposure) and essential service workers (education workers, police officers, firefighters, and military personnel). Within the vulnerable groups, people who reside or work in long-stay establishments for the elderly, people deprived of liberty, and people in shelters or other closed establishments were considered. The average age of the deceased in Uruguay is 76.4 years and a median of 79. It is also found that the prevalence of comorbidities that increase mortality is higher in people over 50 (Ministerio de Salud Pública - Uruguay, 2021b, April).

Vaccination advanced successfully in this first stage, which included all groups of people over 18 years of age.

As of June 2021, vaccination of young people between 12 and 17 years of age began (Uruguay Presidencia, 2021b) and on January 12, children between 5 and 11 years of age were included (Ministerio de Salud Pública 2021h, December).

Communication strategy of vaccination

As mentioned above, the vaccination strategy has a solid base in the government's communication strategy that has sought to build trust based on the value of transparency. Below is an analysis of the communication strategy developed by Schroeder (2022), and now the information collected is expanded and completed.

The Ministry of Public Health's website gained superb visibility during the pandemic and is today the page with the most views within the Executive Branch.

There is another aspect, which perhaps goes unnoticed by the public, that is, the Ministry of Public Health has intensively developed its own social media channels. Thus, it has deepened the work on existing networks such as Facebook, Twitter, and YouTube, and developed Instagram, and recently it is working on Tik Tok and Linkedin.

With a strategy that involves developing appropriate content for each social media, the website of the Ministry of Public Health is the government website with the most visits and its social media channels have grown exponentially in the past 18 months.

The previous work that allowed the development of the digital communication channels of the Ministry of Public Health was undoubtedly an important point of support for the communication strategy of Covid-19.

Table 1 shows the exponential growth of followers in the ministry's social media, which demonstrates an increase in the scope of communication. At the same time, it shows the response of public opinion to the content that is published. It also means that official sources have proved to be reliable for different audiences.

Table 1. Number of followers in social media of the Ministry of Public Health from February 2020 to October 2021

Followers monthly growth MSP

	YouTube		Facebook		Instagram		Twitter		Total
February	1.797		40.410				22.313		64.520
March	2.125	25%	56.640	29%			61.313	74%	120.079
April	8.002	377%	138.000	244%	25.094		73.813	20%	244.915
May	8.425	5%	146.641	6%	33.407	25%	78.787	6%	267.260
June	8.497	1%	148.669	1%	40.930	23%	80.200	2%	278.296
July	8.535	0,5%	152.501	4%	42.150	3%	83.300	4%	286.486
August	8.665	1,5%	154.869	6%	51.679	23%	85.300	2%	300.513
September	8.728	1,0%	156.287	1%	55.557	10%	86.752	1%	307.324
October	9.063	3%	158.489	1%	60.088	11%	88.436	1%	316.076
November	9.240	2%	164.211	4%	64.242	7%	91.043	3%	328.736
December	9.540	3%	171.610	4%	74.351	14%	95.524	5%	351.025
January 2021	9.612	1%	176.831	3%	80.333	7%	98.300	3%	365.076
February	9.737	1%	181.363	3%	84.878	5%	100.775	3%	376.753
March	10.300	6%	197.470	9%	95.799	13%	113.583	13%	417.152
April	10.800	5%	211.731	7%	101.379	5%	122.695	7%	446.605
May	11.200	4%	217.415	3%	105.813	4%	128.325	4%	462.753
June	12.000	1%	222.739	2%	109.238	3%	132.234	3%	476.211
July	12.500	4%	225.588	1%	111.298	2%	135.325	2%	484.711
August	12.900	3%	228.090	1%	112.633	1%	138.483	2%	492.106
September	13.200	2%	229.365	1%	113.143	1%	140.383	2%	496.091
October	13.400	2%	229.803	1%	114.573	1%	143.277	2%	501.053
November	13.600	2%	227.918	-1%	114.738	1%	144.867	1%	501.123
December	13.700	2%	228.276	1%	114.931	1%	146.933	1%	503.840
January 2022	13.800	1%	230.466	1%	118.427	3%	151.358	3%	514.051
February	13.900	1%	231.175	1%	120.026	1%	155.780	3%	520.881
March	13.900	0%	231.195	1%	120.340	1%	158.863	2%	524.298
April	14.024	0,90%	231.349	0%	120.400	0%	161.711	2%	527.484
May	14.088	0,45%	231.839	0,20%	120.938	0,40%	164.728	2%	531.593
Accumulated growth		784%		574%		482%		738%	824%

Communication in social media is combined with public communication of authorities, news in the print media, official releases, and advertisements, among others. Following the definition provided by Coffman (2002, p. 2).

> Public communication campaigns use the media, messaging, and an organized set of communication activities to generate specific outcomes in a large number of individuals and in a specified period of time. They are an attempt to shape behavior toward desirable social outcomes. To maximize their chances of success, campaigns usually coordinate media efforts with a mix of other interpersonal and community-based communication channels.

The author highlights two types of campaigns that seek individual behavioral change or promote behaviors leading to improved individual or social well-being, and public campaigns that try to mobilize society to bring about policy change.

The Covid-19 campaign had a double component. On the one hand, the campaign was a call to action, and, on the other hand, it sought to impose the concept of vaccination as an act of solidarity.

Undoubtedly, in this sense, the Covid-19 vaccination campaign strongly marked Uruguayan society. The country proved to be an example of rapid vaccination and also showed results of vaccination effectiveness. A negative epidemiological situation was reversed (Figure 3), and the economic activity shows a clear improvement.

To be effective, health communication campaigns must take into account the conceptual frameworks mentioned above. The following aspects stand out from the aforementioned theories:

(1) Information should be clear, understandable and impactful.
(2) Communication must be timely and promptly.
(3) The audience's perception of risk and its context (in this case the evolution of the pandemic) must be taken into account.
(4) Knowledge is a relevant factor in health decision-making.
(5) The influence of close groups is also relevant in health decision-making.

Concerning the Covid-19 vaccination strategy in Uruguay, communication had a central place and throughout the process we sought to maintain the trust of the population. The central value is transparency, as it has been throughout the Covid-19 communication (Schroeder & Amadeo, 2021).

A 360° government communication was developed where all communication formats were taken into account to make as much information available to the population as possible.

The following issues are the main aspects of the communication strategy and its implementation on digital platforms.

The website

The Ministry of Public Health´s website is the most visited site among state agencies (Figure 6). During the pandemic and later in the vaccination campaign, it played a fundamental role and the communication team paid special attention to ensure that the information was organized and easily accessible.

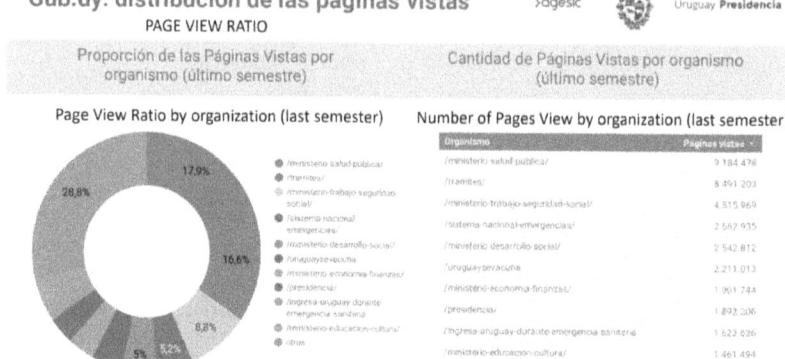

Figure 6. Page view ratio of Ministry of Public Health Site. From: Agencia de gobierno electrónico y Sociedad de la información y conocimiento (n.d.). In this figure it is described the government's page view ratio (Gub.uy), the page view ratio by organization and the number of pages view by organization in the last semester, June 2022.

First of all, a sub-home with relevant information on Covid-19 was organized. The following information was highlighted:

(1) Covid-19 case monitor.
(2) Announcements.
(3) Regulations in force.
(4) News.
(5) Reports.
(6) When the vaccination campaign started, a sub-home with information on the vaccination schedule was developed.
(7) Questions and answers about vaccination.
(8) Questions and answers about vaccines.
(9) Vaccine monitor that allowed seeing the progress of vaccination.
(10) Access to the vaccination certificate.

As of December 2021, the restrictions for entering the country are repealed and entry requirements are established for people with vaccination or without full vaccination. In that instance, this information is prioritized.

Evidence-based communication

Throughout the vaccination process, scientific information was made available to the population in an accessible way in relation to the different vaccine platforms, expected adverse effects of vaccines, questions and answers about vaccines, safety and efficacy of vaccines, effectiveness studies to be carried out, availability of vaccines, and a vaccine monitor that allowed everyone to see the progress of vaccination and its impact on pandemic mitigation.

The communication effort was focused on finding messages in accessible language and the search of interlocutors valued by society. An example of this was the campaign developed with football players where they explained with football metaphors the data on the effectiveness of vaccines.

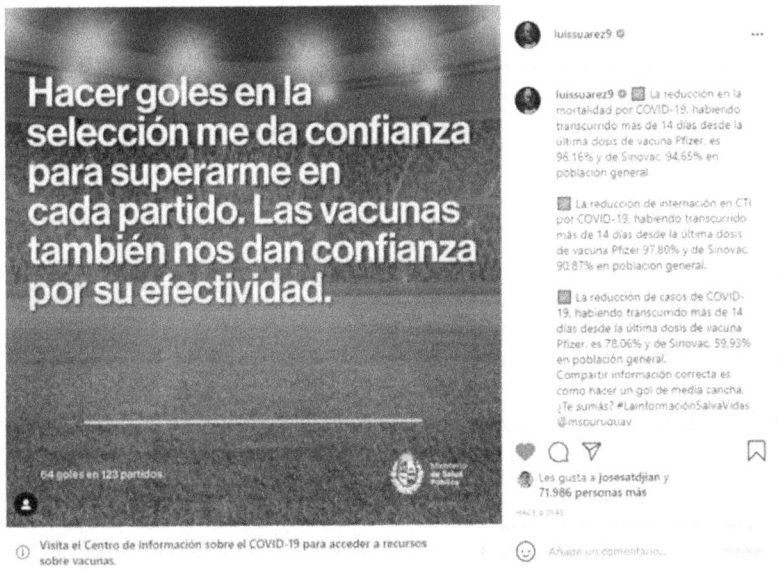

Figure 7. Example of a vaccine effectiveness campaign explained with football metaphors (Luis Suárez). In this example, the text means: "Scoring goals in the National Team gives me confidence to improve myself in each game. Vaccines also give us confidence because of their effectiveness". From News "Science in Football Key" by the Ministerio de Salud Pública – Uruguay, 2021d.

Development of audiovisual contents

Audiovisual contents played an important role in the strategy. For instance, short videos were developed throughout the process to explain synthetically some relevant aspects of vaccination.

Experts, doctors, and nurses were sought to develop the vaccination program message clearly. The principal concepts developed in the vaccination campaign were as follows: Uruguay has always had high vaccination rates; vaccines are safe; they are the main tool to get out of this long process that affected all of us; they were developed in record time under exceptional circumstances and with a collaborative process of government and science; and self-care must be maintained for the vaccines to be effective.

Infographics developments

Infographics were developed to explain in a simple way very complex concepts such as those related to the effectiveness of vaccination. These materials were disseminated in social media channels of the Ministry of Public Health and had a high impact on the public opinion. This information was also taken by local news and the main press, and it was widely disseminated. Simplifying a complex message allows it to have a greater reach.

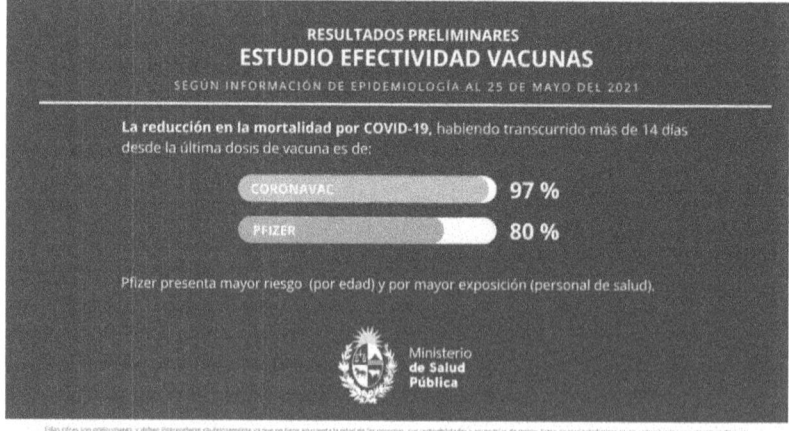

Figure 8. Infographic on the effectiveness of Covid-19 vaccines. From "Estudio sobre efectividad vacunal" by Dirección del Departamento de Vigilancia en Salud Ministerio de Salud Pública – Uruguay, 2021c.

#UruguaySeVacuna

The hashtag of the campaign was #UruguaySeVacuna and had great repercussions. A global phenomenon to which Uruguay was no stranger was the photo of the moment of vaccination, with the vaccinators, at the vaccinator's office and with messages expressing solidarity: "I am getting vaccinated for me, for my family, for my loved ones".

People from the world of art and sports, journalists, religious leaders, politicians, and others showed their support for the vaccination campaign. Social media allowed to show the images of hundreds of social referents, and this not only favored the amplification of the message but also collaborated in the contagion effect.

Combating misinformation

As already stated, the pandemic brought misinformation as a collateral effect. Globally, the most common false claims are that the vaccine modifies the human genome or implants tracking chips, induces damage to health or contains human immunodeficiency virus particles. These false statements are also related to messages regarding the denial of the pandemic and that it is not necessary to use protective measures such as the use of masks (Rzymski, P., Borkowski, L., Drąg, M., Flisiak, R., Jemielity, J., Krajewski, J., Mastalerz-Migas, A., et al. 2021).

Among the deniers, there is a subgroup of anti-vaccers that also have a global presence and Uruguay was not alien to this phenomenon. These anti-vaccers groups promote messages mainly on the social network Facebook, Twitter, and Telegram. However, the local media did not give them relevant coverage, and the social demonstrations were of little impact.

Because it is a global phenomenon and it can potentially negatively impact, it had to be monitored by the communication team of the Ministry of Public Health. This is the first misinformation phenomenon that the country has experienced on a large scale. Likewise, Uruguay is characterized by having reliable and impartial information media. Consequently, it coins freedom of press and is one of the main strengths of the democratic system.

It is noteworthy that the media throughout the pandemic cited as their main sources of information the content provided by the Ministry of Public Health and the Presidency of the Republic. This fact shows that trust in official sources has been maintained from the beginning of the pandemic to date. This is a positive consequence of the communication policy based on transparency promoted by President Lacalle Pou.

To have a better understanding of the subject, the Ministry of Public Health commissioned the consulting firm Civirt to conduct an analysis of misinformation on social media. The study consisted of fan analysis on Twitter identifying the nodes of disinformation and their followers during February 10 to March 10, 2021. Fifteen were detected and within this group four with greater activity. Moreover, the Facebook page that is cited by these users as a source of content was also analyzed.

The study concludes that the most repeated lies on social media are five:

1. There is an epidemic of false positives, and tests performed with the PCR diagnostic technique are not reliable.
2. Vaccines are not safe.
3. Deaths from Covid-19 are fewer than reported.
4. Mouthpieces are not necessary as they are harmful.
5. Vaccines are not effective.

Based on this analysis, the communication strategy focused on reinforcing the information about the questioned aspects. The Ministry did not seek a form of confrontation or debate with the anti-vaccine movements but rather reinforced the information in relation to the safety, efficacy, and effectiveness of the vaccine.

Mainly, it was sought to disseminate effectiveness studies that were developed very early by the Ministry of Public Health. These studies were shown through videos and infographics with the purpose of having the widest possible reach. In this regard, the amplification by the authorities (Minister and Undersecretary) were highly positive. Fundamentally, the Twitter account of Minister Salinas has a relevant scope. Salinas has the particularity of interacting personally with users, and this led to building trust with the public opinion and journalists. In addition, vaccine effectiveness studies were widely disseminated by referents of the scientific community, doctors, and scientists who have a high reputation in Uruguay. This last aspect also contributed to reinforce trust.

Development of rational messaging

The campaign had a strong emphasis on rational messages and communication based on scientific evidence. This format was prioritized in order to provide as much information as possible about the vaccination process, vaccines, the functioning of the schedule, among others (Ministerio de Salud Pública – Uruguay, 2021b, 2021g).

The content of the messages is summarized in the following concepts:

(1) Vaccination will be free and not mandatory.
(2) Vaccine doses are sufficient to achieve herd immunity.
(3) Vaccination is an act of solidarity, and it is necessary to be vaccinated to stop the pandemic.
(4) It will be carried out in a staggered manner, according to prioritized groups.
(5) The dates when people will receive the vaccine are reported to be the website, Coronavirus app, and call centers are promoted as the main means of communication.
(6) It is necessary to maintain personal care while progressing with the vaccination plan.
(7) The different groups that should be scheduled to receive the vaccine are announced in stages.

Final conclusions

The Covid-19 vaccination plan is about to end, and the set objectives have been achieved. The first objective was 70 % of the target population and then that objective was increased to 80 % of the total population of the country.

Uruguay achieved a high vaccination rate and the expected health objectives were achieved: fewer infections, fewer seriously hospitalized patients and, consequently, fewer deaths (Figure 4).

Both the President of the Republic and the Minister of Public Health have a high rate of approval regarding the management of the pandemic (El 84 % de la población aprueba la gestión de la pandemia realizada por Lacalle, según Factum. [84 % of the Population Approves Lacalle's Handling of the Pandemic, According to Factum.], 2021). The Minister of Public Health is the minister with the highest popular approval (Cifra, 2021).

This data reveals the high level of confidence acquired in the past 18 months of government management. In this critical phase of the pandemic, public opinion verified that the established objectives were met, an orderly vaccination was developed, and all the people who wanted to be vaccinated were able to do so. The data also showed that the vaccines are safe and effective. In general, communication was an essential issue of a very good government management, particularly digital communication was necessary to achieve an effective campaign.

Confidence in the government resulted in an excellent response from the population and other social actors such as opinion leaders, leaders from the scientific world, businessmen, among others.

The government communication strategy occupied a predominant place, before vaccination and during vaccination. A communication management based on transparency and an appeal to responsible freedom had a positive response from the population. In the first phase, the population showed a high level of compliance with the non-pharmacological measures promoted to deal with the pandemic, and in the vaccination phase, there was a positive attitude that resulted in a rapid advance in vaccination.

A future analysis is pending to understand the reasons that led people to get vaccinated with an emergency vaccine. Questions remain, especially about some groups that are of interest for future public vaccination policies: how was the decision process for children (which motivated their parents to vaccinate or not vaccinate them) and young people.

Bibliography

Ajzen, I. (1985). "From Intentions to Actions: A Theory of Planned Behavior", in *Action Control*, Kuhl and J. Keckmann (eds.), 11–39. Springer, Berlin.

Bandura, A. (1997). *Self-Efficacy: The Exercise of Control*. Freeman, New York.

Becker, M. H., Haefner, D. P., and Maiman, L. A. (1977). "The health belief model in the prediction of dietary compliance: A field experiment", in *Journal of Health and Social Behaviour*, 18, 348–366.

Cacioppo, J. and Petty, R. (1984). "The elaboration likelihood model of persuasion", *in NA - Advances in Consumer Research* (vol. 11) T. C. Kinnear (ed.), 673–675. Association for Consumer Research. https://www.acrwebsite.org/volumes/6329/volumes/v11/NA%20-%2011

Cifra. (2021). *Evaluación de la Gestión de Ministros*. https://www.cifra.com.uy/index.php/2021/08/10/evaluacion-de-la-gestion-de-ministros-3/

Coffman, J. (2002). *Public Communication Campaign Evaluation: An Environmental Scan of Challenges, Criticisms, Practice, and Opportunities.* Communications Consortium Media Center https://www.dors.it/documentazione/testo/200905/Public%20Communication%20Campaign%20Evaluation.pdf

Figueroa, M. E., Kincaid, D. L., Rani, M., and Lewis, G. (2002). *Communication for Social Change: An Integrated Model for Measuring the Process and Its Outcomes.* Rockefeller: Foundation and Johns Hopkins University Center for Communication Programs.

González-Melado, F. J., and Di Pietro, M. L. (2020). La vacuna frente al Covid-19 y la confianza institucional. *Enfermedades Infecciosas y Microbiología Clínica.* https://doi.org/10.1016/j.eimc.2020.08.001

Janz, N. K., and Becker, M. H. (1984). "The health belief model: A decade later", in *Health Education Quarterly*, 11 (1), 1–47.

Kincaid, D. L. (1979). *The Convergence Model of Communication.* EastWest Communication Institute, Australia.

Ministerio de Salud Pública – Uruguay (2021a, March 1). *Plan de vacunación contra COVID-19: Responsabilidad cívica y solidaria.* https://www.gub.uy/ministerio-salud-publica/comunicacion/noticias/plan-vacunacion-contra-covid-19-responsabilidad-civica-solidaria

Ministerio de Salud Pública – Uruguay (2021b April, 15). *Plan Estratégico de Vacunación covid-19.* https://www.gub.uy/ministerio-salud-publica/comunicacion/noticias/plan-estrategico-vacunacion-contra-covid-19

Ministerio de Salud Pública – Uruguay (2021c, May 27). *Estudio sobre efectividad vacunal.* https://www.gub.uy/ministerio-salud-publica/comunicacion/noticias/estan-disponibles-datos-preliminares-del-estudio-efectividad-vacunal

Ministerio de Salud Pública – Uruguay (2021d, July 12). *Ciencia en clave de fútbol.* https://www.gub.uy/ministerio-salud-publica/comunicacion/noticias/campana-efectividad-vacunal-ciencia-clave-futbol

Ministerio de Salud Pública – Uruguay (2021f, November 1). *Monitor de datos de vacunación Covid-19.* https://monitor.uruguaysevacuna.gub.uy/

Ministerio de Salud Pública – Uruguay (2021g, February 26). *Campaña de vacunación COVID-19 #UruguaySeVacuna*. [Videos]. YouTube. https://www.youtube.com/playlist?list=PL4O9exeLSKwyeofFVi_3x3Vqcl1gZ-6Qa

Ministerio de Salud Pública – Uruguay (2021h, December 29*). En enero comienza la vacunación contra covid-19 en niños entre 5 y 11 años.* https://www.gub.uy/ministerio-salud-publica/comunicacion/noticias/enero-comienza-vacunacion-contra-covid-ninos-entre-5-11-anos#:~:text=La%20agenda%20para%20solicitar%20d%C3%ADa,12%20de%20enero%20del%202022.

Ministerio de Salud Pública – Uruguay (2022a, January 12). Inmunización contra covid en niños comenzó hoy, con la inauguración de un nuevo vacunatorio en el Pereira Rossel. https://www.gub.uy/ministerio-salud-publica/comunicacion/noticias/enero-comienza-vacunacion-contra-covid-ninos-entre-5-11-anos.

Ministerio de Salud Pública – Uruguay (2022b, May 30). *Informe epidemiológico COVID-19 Actualización al 21 de mayo de 2022.* https://www.gub.uy/ministerio-salud-publica/comunicacion/noticias/informe-epidemiologico-covid-19-actualizado-18-enero-2021

Ministerio de Salud Pública – Uruguay. [@MSPURUGUAY]. (2021g, January 5). En comparencia ante la Comisión de Salud Pública del @SenadoUy, el ministro @DrDanielSalinas explicó el trabajo realizado desde marzo hasta la fecha. [Image attached] [Tweet]. Twitter. https://twitter.com/MSPUruguay/status/1346539663104888833

Miranda criticó la lentitud del gobierno y dijo que es necesario tomar medidas urgentes. El presidente del Frente Amplio dijo además que el partido tiene numerosos vínculos para acelerar la llegada de la vacuna si es necesario. (2021, December 14). *El País.* https://www.elpais.com.uy/informacion/politica/miranda-critico-lentitud-gobierno-dijo-necesario-tomar-medidas-urgentes.html

Montagni, I., Ouazzani-Touhami, K., Mebarki, A., Texier, N., Schück, S., and Tzourio, C. (2021). "Acceptance of a Covid-19 vaccine is associated with ability to detect fake news and health literacy", *Journal of Public Health*. 10.1093/pubmed/fdab028

Moreno, A. R., y Peres, F. (2020). Comunicación de riesgos ante el Coronavirus. *Boletín sobre COVID-19*, 1(4), 7–9.

Moya, M. (2000). "Persuasión y cambio de actitudes", in *Psicología social*, J. F. Morales and C. Huici (coords.), UNED, Madrid, pp. 153–170.

Nespereira, J. (2014). *Estrategias discursivas en la comunicación de crisis sanitarias (retórica y teoría de la argumentación): el caso de la gripe A en 2009* (Tesis Doctoral, Universidad de Valladolid). Teseo. https://www.educacion.gob.es/teseo/mostrarSeleccion.do

Oreggiani, I. (2015). *El camino hacia la cobertura universal en Uruguay: cobertura poblsvionsl del Sistema Nacional Integrado de Salud*. Organización Panamericana de la salud: https://www.paho.org/es/documentos/avances-consolidacion-sistema-nacional-integrado-salud Pan American Health Organization (2021). *Guía para elaborar una estrategia de comunicación de riesgos sobre las vacunas contra la COVID-19*. https://iris.paho.org/handle/10665.2/53259

Petty, R. E. and Cacioppo, J. T. (1986). "The elaboration likelihood mode of persuasion", in *Communication and Persuasión: Central and Peripheral Routes to Attitude Change*, New York, NY: Springer, 1–24.

Rogers, E. M. (1995). *Diffusion of Innovations*. (4th ed.). Free Press, New York.

Rogers, E. M. and Kincaid, D. L. (1981). *Communication Networks: Towards a New Paradigm for Research*. Free Press, New York.

Roozenbeek, J., Schneider, C. R., Dryhurst, S., Kerr, J., Freeman, A. L., Recchia, G., van der Bles, A. M. and van der Linden, S. (2020). "Susceptibility to misinformation about COVID-19 around the world", in *Royal Society Open Science*, 7 (10),. https://royalsocietypublishing.org/doi/full/10.1098/rsos.201199

Rosenstock, I. M., Strecher, V. J., and Becker, M. H. (1988). "Social learning theory and the health belief model", in *Health Education Quarterly*, 15 (2), 175–183.

Rzymski, P., Borkowski, L., Drąg, M., Flisiak, R., Jemielity, J., Krajewski, J., Mastalerz-Migas, A., Mastalerz-Migas, A., Matyja, A., Pyrc, K., Simon, K., Sutkowski, M., Wysocki, J., Zajkowska, J., and Fal, A. (2021). "The strategies to support the COVID-19 vaccination with evidence-based communication and tackling misinformation", In *Vaccines*, 9 (2), 109. https://www.mdpi.com/2076-393X/9/2/109

Schiavo, R. (2013). *Health Communication: From Theory to Practice* (Vol. 217). John Wiley & Sons, San Francisco.

Schroeder, P. (2022). "Covid-19 vaccination campaign: The uruguayan case-contributions of digital communication", in *Navigating Digital Communication and Challenges for Organizations*, J. Andrade, and T. Ruão (eds.), 93–112. IGI Ed. https://doi.org/Doi:10.4018/978-1-7998-9790-3.ch006.

Schroeder, P. and Amadeo, B. (2021). "Communication strategy for COVID-19 in Uruguay", in *Strategic Communication in Context: Theoretical Debates and Applied Research*, S. Balonas, T. Ruão T. and M. C. Carrillo (eds.), 295–322. UMinho Editora. https://doi.org/10.21814/uminho.ed.46.13

Schwarzinger, M. and Luchini, S. (2021). "Addressing COVID-19 vaccine hesitancy: Is official communication the key?", *The Lancet Public Health*, 6 (6), e353–e354.

Storlie, C. B., Pollock, B. D. Rojas, R. L., Demuth, G. O., Johnson, P. W., Wilson, P. M., Heinzen, E. P., Liu, H., Carter, R. E., Habermann, E. B., Kor, D. J., Neville, M. R., Limper, A. H., Noe, K. H., Bydon, M., Franco, P. M., Sampathkumar, P., Shah, N. D., Dunlay, S. M. and Dowdy, S. C. (2021). "Quantifying the importance of COVID-19 vaccination to our future outlook", in *Mayo Clinic Proceedings*, 96 (7), 1890–1895. https://doi.org/10.1016/j.mayocp.2021.04.012

Strecher, V. J. and Rosenstock, I. M. (1997). *The Health Belief Model*. Jossey-Bass.

Strecher, V. J., McEvoy DeVellis, B., Becker, M. H. and Rosenstock, I. M. (1986). "The role of self-efficacy in achieving health behavior change" in *Health Education Quarterly*, 13(1), 73–92. https://doi.org/10.1177/109019818601300108

Tench R. and Bridge G. (2021). "Developing effective health communication campaigns", in *Strategic Communication in Context: Theoretical Debates and Applied Research*, S. Balonas, T. Ruão T. & M. C. Carrillo (eds.), 69–86. UMinho Editora. https://doi.org/10.21814/uminho.ed.46.4

Tormo, M. J., & Banegas, J. R. (2001). "Mejorar la comunicación de riesgos en Salud Pública: sin tiempo para demoras", in *Revista Española de Salud Pública*, 75(1), 00. http://scielo.isciii.es/scielo.php?script=sci_arttext&pid=S1135-57272001000100001&lng=es&tlng=es.

Uruguay Presidencia. (2021a, January 23). *Gobierno adquirió 3,75 millones de vacunas contra la COVID-19 y aspira a inocular a 2,8 millones de personas*. https://www.gub.uy/presidencia/comunicacion/noticias/gobierno-adquirio-375-millones-vacunas-contra-covid-19-aspira-inocular-28

Uruguay Presidencia (2021b, June 9). *Comenzó la vacunación de menores de18 años con 157.000 jóvenes inscriptos.* https://www.gub.uy/presidencia/comunicacion/noticias/comenzo-vacunacion-menores-18-anos-157000-jovenes-inscriptos

Uruguay XXI. (2021, Juanuary 2nd). *Uruguay es el mejor de América en la gestión de la pandemia.* https://www.uruguayxxi.gub.uy/es/noticias/articulo/uruguay-es-el-mejor-de-america-en-gestion-de-la-pandemia/

Vacunas: el FA suma presión al gobierno con nuevas críticas por falta de transparencia. (2021, February 19). *El Observador.* https://www.elobservador.com.uy/nota/frente-amplio-vuelve-a-la-carga-por-las-vacunas-y-reclama-por-su-llegada-202121817480

World Health Organization. (2022). WHO SAGE values framework for the allocation and prioritization of COVID-19 vaccionatrion, 14 September, 2020.!https://apps.who.int/iris/handle/10665/334299?locale-attribute=en&

[1] Pandemic mitigation, in terms of health strategy, involves reduction of infections, severe cases and mortality.

The challenge of higher education through virtual education platforms during Covid-19: The Peruvian case

Mariana Nicolini Zevallos – *Universidad Peruana de Ciencias Aplicadas*

Giancarlo Gomero – *Universidad Peruana de Ciencias Aplicadas*

Introduction

Covid-19 is a disease caused by the coronavirus known as SARS-CoV-2 (WHO 2020). The virus is highly contagious and is transmitted from person to person by coughing or respiratory secretions. The virus spread around the world in a very accelerated manner (Gastelo, Maguiña & Tequen 2020: 125), thus becoming the most important global health emergency since 1920 with the Spanish flu (Cabezas, Castro, Chowell, Cornejo, Garro, Ibarguen, La Torre Rosillo, Loayza, Mezarina, Mimbela, Munayco, Ordinola, Quijano, Ramos, Reyes, Rojas-Vasquez, Rothenberg, Soto-Cabeza, Tariq, Valle, 2020: 339). By January 24, 2020, the virus, born in China, had already spread to other cities in that country, raising the number of infected people to 835 (Gastelo, Maguiña & Tequen 2020: 125). At the same time it was spreading globally and was declared a pandemic by the World Health Organization (WHO) on March 11, 2020 (WHO 2021). In Peru, the first case was registered on March 6, and on March 11 the country declared a Health Emergency for 90 days (Miyahira 2020:83). Inequality exacerbated a pre-existing educational crisis, as the pandemic destabilized education systems worldwide (UNESCO, 2021).

In these circumstances, teachers of all sectors and levels have had to adapt to the situation, going through challenges they were not used to in their regular professional practice, having to move from face-to-face to virtual teaching (Carabelli 2020: 189). This adaptation for online teaching is linked to the mental health of the teachers themselves (Bravo, Reynosa, Rivera, & Rodríguez 2020: 142). Therefore, it is important to mention that teachers show different perspectives and experiences regarding educational technologies, where some see these processes in an optimistic way and others do not (Albuquerque, Arteaga, Costas, Muñoz, Porta, Sunday, Tomczyk, Yasar 2021: 2739). Likewise, one of the transcendental challenges that teachers have had to face in virtual education is connectivity (Barrios, Delgado, Maradey 2021: 142). In the Peruvian context, connectivity is linked to acute socio-economic and opportunity inequalities (Expósito & Marsollier 2020: 19). In these circumstances, the teaching role must respond to the challenges presented and manage the use of digital materials and the application of teaching and assessment strategies, implementing a model of actions for this purpose (Agudelo 2009: 120).

In the midst of this health emergency, the use of virtual education platforms was necessary, these being fundamental tools for distance education (Palma, Romero, Soledispa, Zuña 2020: 353) useful for imparting knowledge and a resource that generates improvement at a cognitive level (Barrera & Guapi 2018). In addition, Anchundia, Arboleda, Astudillo and Pinto (2018: 591) point out that these platforms generate a teacher–student approach, which promotes and stimulates socialization. In its beginnings, online teaching had a scheme very similar to traditional teaching, but as the years went by, educational training was updated and improved *ad hoc* to this model with the development of digital didactic materials, in this case virtual education platforms (Wang, Zhang & Zhou 2020: 162831), at the same time increasing student satisfaction within the course (Benta, Bologa & Dzita 2014: 1171). The platforms also favor the creation of virtual environments, allowing autonomous and flexible student learning (Gil, Montoya & Sepúlveda 2019: 2 and Barrios, Delgado, Maradey 2021: 143). With a good organization of the subjects they can enrich and promote learning (Vargas & Villalobos 2018: 23), being of great help for the immediate and flexible approach of the student, in terms of location and time (Carretero & Hermosilla 2004: 141).

As it has a significant impact on teachers both positively and negatively (Hernández, Loor, Palma & Salazar 2021: 97), it is necessary for them to have continuous training (Cotohuanca, 2021:132). Despite the abrupt change, teachers had to comply with the curricular objectives and their technological knowledge has been key to this, also requiring that students, at the same time, develop critical and reflective thinking in this environment (Cervi, Parola, Tejedor & Tusa 2020: 22) since teaching standards, in terms of quality and content, have not changed (López, 2020: 3). Thus, pedagogical quality and good teacher preparation with the use of ICTs facilitate and improve teaching in addition to favoring their own adaptation to transfer their knowledge to students (Juca 2016: 107). Ara, Magaña, Mendoza, San Román and Yepez (2019: 12) mention that the use of ICTs has become part of the daily life of teachers and students, being indispensable for the educational process, so their use should be encouraged (Viñas 2017: 157).

Media literacy is a broad and complex image of ideas, and with a diversity of interpretations, this occurs due to the accelerated growth of its conceptual application in pedagogical processes, which generates a growing academic interest (Potter 2010: 675). Aguaded (2012: 7) and Jooyeun (2017: 6) analyze media literacy from different points of view, while for the former this is characterized by making use of the digital environment to develop our different competencies with critical thinking, which becomes a right of every person; for the latter this is rather the way that allows us to interact with the digital world through different forms of communication giving us the possibility to develop ourselves at our choice, comparing information and being able to transmit it. Thus, Aufderheide (1993) describes media literacy as the ability of people to access information, then analyze and evaluate it, and finally communicating the message in different ways. Hence both the media and the way they present their messages are constantly updated (Potter 2010: 682) so that obtaining knowledge occurs continuously, confirming the urgency to master certain languages, as they exist within technology (Herrera, Pinto, Valdivia 2018: 3). All this encompasses more and more presence in higher education, since the objective of media literacy is to empower the one who uses technology permanently and, at the same time, that this acquires knowledge about the media to then create and distribute content (UN, 2020).

Lázaro-Cantabrana, Silva and Usart (2019: 34) point out that the development of digital competencies in teachers should begin with their initial training and continue throughout their careers. Similarly, Cisneros-Cohernour, Cordero, Espinosa, García, Ponce and Serrano, (2018: 346) and Cabero and Palacios (2021: 179) highlight that the development of these competencies such as organization, understanding, patience, etc., promote the feedback of student performance and boost it emotionally and socially; designing and enhancing the teaching-learning process, building relationships on both sides. This is also where the media competencies developed by teachers can be observed. Ferrés and Piscitelli (2012: 79) and Jooyeun (2017: 10) define it in different ways: the first mention the mastery of skills, knowledge and attitudes with basic dimensions, without guaranteeing good professional performance, but the improvement with respect to a given skill; and the second refers to the mastery of knowledge, skills and attitudes in the field of participation both as people who receive messages and interact with them and as people who produce messages, allowing them to orient themselves in a mediatized world and actively know it with the help of the media.

This research proposes to analyze the preparation of higher education teachers regarding the use of virtual education platforms and their impact after the Covid-19 pandemic, and to analyze the competencies acquired by teachers in relation to these platforms. This seeks to recognize the particularities in the perceptions of teachers regarding the training and learning processes, which were accelerated due to the urgency of the pandemic to generate a response and that each one experienced differently either by the strategies taken or by their own previous capacities, all to overcome the situation and achieve their objectives.

We will work with the following categories and subcategories:

(1) Previous characteristics of teachers
(2) Use of virtual education platforms.
(3) Media literacy.
(4) Adaptation and training of teachers.
(5) Media competition.
(6) Development of educational digital competencies.

These categories are related to the specific objectives:

(1) Examine the use of virtual education platforms.
(2) To explore the acquired competencies of higher education teachers during the use of virtual education platforms.

We answer our specific questions:

(1) How do teachers interact within the virtual education platforms?
(2) What are the new competencies acquired from the continuous use of virtual education platforms by teachers?

The area of study to which our research belongs is that of communication and education, as well as the interaction with new media in and for education. This helps to understand the state in which teachers are, their adaptation and what they need to improve their teaching methodology, as well as their developed media competencies and how they use them during teaching.

Methodology

To conduct this research we started from an interpretative paradigm González- Monteagudo (2001: 228), we interpreted and analyzed what was described by the participants during the research and this was adapted to reality according to their own progress and data collection (Flick 2015). Likewise, we respond to a phenomenological study design where the nature of the lived experiences is recognized in relation to a phenomenon or fact and the meaning given by those involved in the research Creswell (2003).

A qualitative approach was adopted (Creswell & Creswell, 2017) given the nature of the data collected, based on opinions, perceptions and points of view. The technique used for the present research was the semi-structured interview, and we found it adequate to be able to respond to the general objective, which was to analyze the preparation that higher education teachers have in virtual education through virtual education platforms during the Covid-19 pandemic. This also includes specific objectives. The interview, according to Kvale (2011), is a data collection technique that is mostly used to learn more about a topic from the point of view of a subject under study, in this case the interviewee being one of the essential approaches in data collection for qualitative research, creating knowledge through the interrelationship between the interviewer and the interviewee. In addition, answers are obtained based on the opinions and experiences of each sample with the possibility of collecting several results (Vargas 2012: 121). In this sense, the interviewer conducts the interview to obtain the reasons or poses critical questions without exposing his own point of view on the subject (Kvale 2011). The instrument used was an interview guide divided into three blocks: media literacy, use of virtual education platforms and media competence. These blocks were divided at the same time into the following categories: previous characteristics of teachers, and adaptation and training of teachers. The instrument was given to two communication and humanities professionals for validation. Observations were collected, and respective changes were made to optimize it.

As for the sample, a convenience sampling was used and helped by a call through the "snowball" technique, that is, some interviewees helped us to reach others with the same characteristics we were looking for. The sample was composed of 10 higher education teachers between 30 and 60 years of age. Five of the interviewees were from the city of Lima, both public and private universities, and the other five were from provinces in the interior of Peru, both public and private universities. Each of the interviewees came from different universities, and we tried to ensure that their teaching specialties were varied and that these were not in the area of communication, considering that their study centers were located in different parts of Peru. In this way we were able to contact professors in the fields of law, chemistry, accounting and psychology. In the beginning, we were able to contact professional colleagues whom we were also able to interview, obtain different opinions and experiences – from different points of view always based on their own experience – and obtain a comparative research. The interviews were conducted between March 24 and March 31, 2021. These were conducted according to the availability of the participants, who were the ones to indicate date and time. All were conducted virtually through the Google Meet platform so that the time could be optimized and not have to make any transfers. With regard to the approach to the results, we based ourselves on the objectives and categorization previously indicated, based on the previous characteristics of the teachers, their adaptation and training during the Covid-19 pandemic and to learn about their experiences in terms of media literacy, the use of virtual education platforms, the skills acquired, the challenges they faced, the methodologies used; as well as to learn about the implications on the subject of evaluations.

Regarding the method of data protection and confidentiality, a document was prepared informing each of the interviewees about the process regarding the confidentiality of the information and their answers. It was made known that the only persons responsible for the information are those involved in the research. Likewise, they were informed that the recorded interviews are exclusively for research purposes. Finally, it was mentioned that what is required is information that does not involve confidential data unrelated to the research. As ethical considerations, they were given written consent in which they attached their name and signature. As for the risks, it should be noted that there were none at the time of participating in this research. In case any interviewee felt uncomfortable with any question, he/she could leave the interview at any time he/she wished. In addition, it was mentioned to them that as a benefit they could obtain the information of the results of the research in a confidential manner.

With respect to data analysis, after conducting all the interviews, the interviews were transcribed and classified according to categories and subcategories that responded to the research objectives and subobjectives. In addition, at the time of classifying the information, some categories emerged that were obtained due to their repetition among the interviewees' answers.

Among the previous characteristics of the teachers, the specialty in which they teach, the type of university and the time they have been teaching were considered. Regarding media literacy, the approach they had with teaching through technological media, how prepared they were to teach classes through virtual education platforms, the first time they taught classes through virtual education platforms and their knowledge about virtual communication platforms were considered. Regarding the use of virtual education platforms, which virtual education platforms are used, the frequency of their use, if they master them, the interaction they perform within the platform, if they feel its use is beneficial and if the platform used allows them to create a link with the students were taken into consideration. Thus, new categories emerged, such as the functions used in the platforms and the organization within the platforms. Within the category of teacher adaptation and training, there was the category of challenges, from which other categories emerged such as distracters, student motivation, evaluations, connectivity and time. In the category of teachers' media competencies and teacher training, as well as extra resources, the category of extra tools emerged, referring to other technological elements that complement the use of the platforms. Finally, the development of competencies and teaching methodology was analyzed.

Results and discussion

After the data collection, an analysis of the responses of higher education teachers about their preparation and adaptation to the use of virtual education platforms during the Covid-19 pandemic was carried out.

Previous characteristics of teachers in terms of media literacy and the use of virtual education platforms

Regarding the previous characteristics of teachers about their media literacy and the use of virtual education platforms, it was observed that there are certain differences among teachers, and these have to do with the type of university in which they teach their classes and the faculty to which they belong. In this sense, teachers from private universities, whether from Lima or the interior of the country, coincide in mentioning that their knowledge about virtual education platforms prior to the pandemic revolved around the use of the Virtual Classroom in each of their universities, in this case they mention Blackboard, as shown in Figure 1 and Moodle as shown in Figure 2, or the university's own websites, i.e. to post attendance, upload notes or share files, but not to teach their class through this medium. Although one teacher mentions that he had previously received training in Microsoft Teams, he had not used it as a teacher either. On the other hand, teachers at public universities differ from each other, since only one of our sample made use of platforms such as the Virtual Classroom. In the case of Sumweb, the public university Federico Villarreal's own platform, two teachers also commented that due to their courses, one related to urban planning and the other to forestry sciences, they worked with different platforms and tools, but they always did it in a face-to-face mode, until before the pandemic.

Another case, pointed out by a teacher, was that the platform was installed in the university but they did not use it because they did not think it was convenient; this was the case of Moodle and two of the teachers detail that they had a very basic knowledge about these platforms, but that they had not used them before the pandemic, perhaps only for a call related to some exception in the course, as is the case of Google Meet. This is confirmed by (Carabelli 2020: 190), when he states that even though virtual education platforms were already available, the Covid-19 pandemic caused them to be massified and discovered, in some cases for the first time. Likewise, teachers at private universities mentioned that they have been using Blackboard or Moodle platforms for several years. However, in the case of teachers from public universities, two say that they started using Moodle in 2018, but the rest had not yet started using it.

Images of the virtual education platforms mostly used by teachers:

Higher education by virtual education in Covid-19

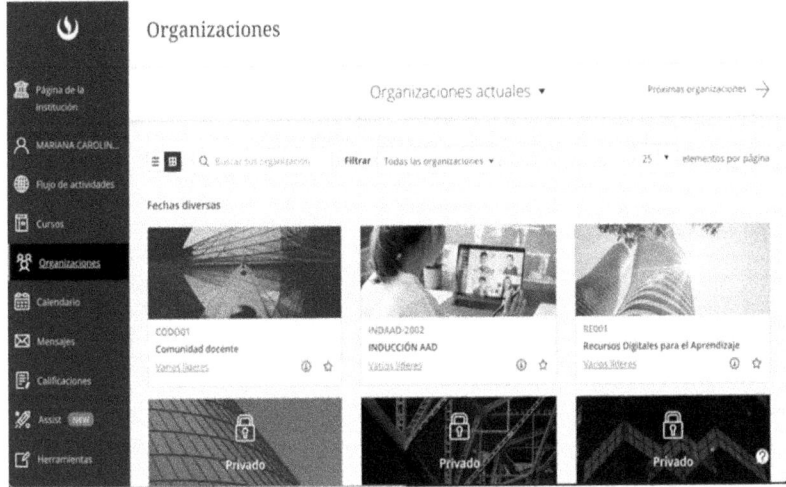

Figure 1. Blackboard Platform.

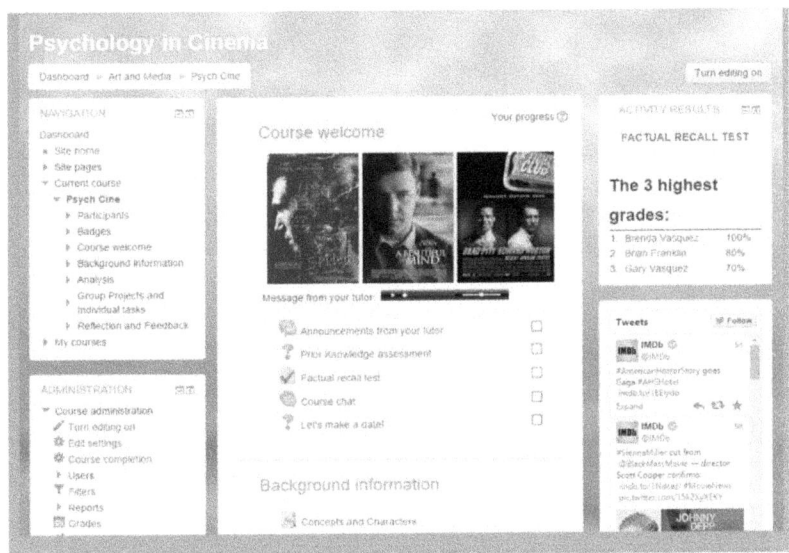

Figure 2. Moodle Platform.

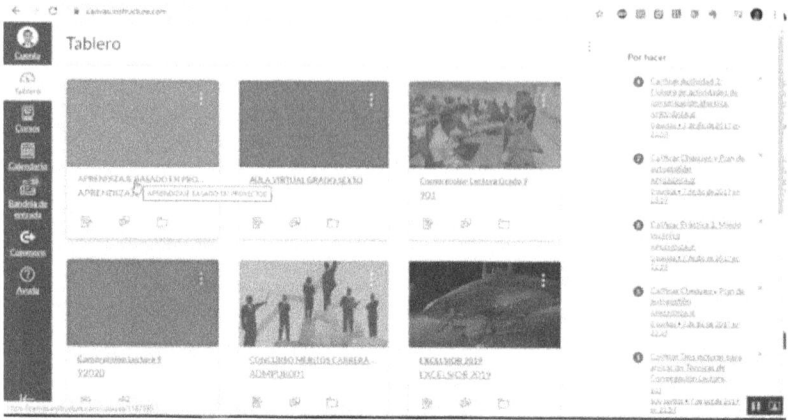

Figure 3. Canvas Platform.

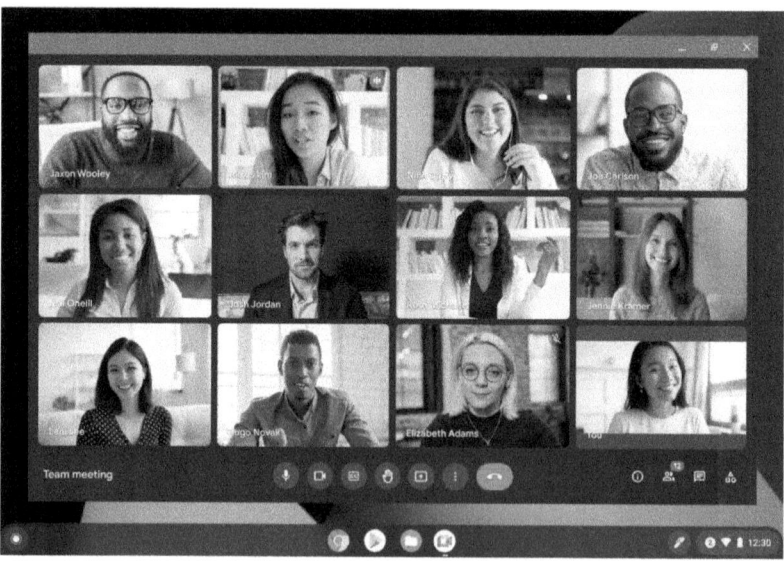

Figure 4. Microsoft Teams Platform.

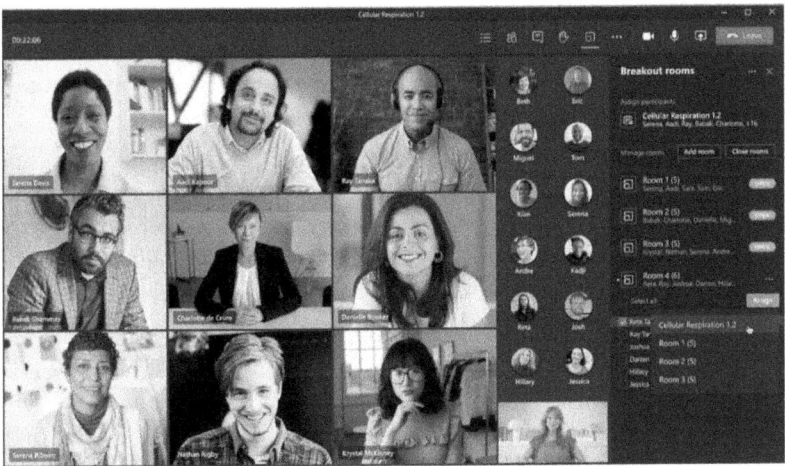

Figure 5. Google Meet Platform.

Adaptation and training of pandemic teachers in the use of virtual education platforms

As for the platforms used by teachers after the pandemic, it varies depending on each teaching center, where Blackboard, Canvas, Moodle, Microsoft Teams and the Zoom platform coupled with another larger platform predominate. However, at the Universidad Nacional Mayor de San Marcos, Google Meet and the Microsoft Teams platform are used. In the case of the Universidad Nacional de Tumbes, a mixture of platforms is used for synchronous sessions in which Cisco Webex, Zoom, Google Meet, Microsoft Teams and Moodle are used for asynchronous sessions. Unlike the rest, a teacher from the Universidad Nacional Agraria La Molina, mentions that she uses the Zoom platform to teach classes, but she uses Google Drive to upload files and so on, because neither she nor her colleagues find the other platforms user-friendly. The teachers mention that at this point, after having been using the platforms since 2020, they consider they have an appropriate management of these platforms to teach their class. Two teachers stand out from our sample, both from Lima but one from a public university and the other from a private university, who mentioned that they do have a command, described as very good, of the virtual education platforms: one of them was helped by having studied distance courses previously, and the other mentions that his extra knowledge in programming and his age are factors that allowed him to manage and master the platforms. In other words, both of them show a good command of the platforms due to knowledge and competencies that are not directly related to teaching activities.

Coinciding with what Barrera and Guapi (2018) state, platforms are tools where knowledge is imparted and improvements can be generated at a cognitive level. Unlike the rest of the teachers, who mention that they will always continue learning and learning utilities within the platforms, even if they already know the basics to teach their sessions. All teachers agree that they spend most of their time during the week on these platforms since they not only use them to teach their classes but also to upload files, notes, coordinate and hold meetings, so they state that their use is constant and that this continuous use saturates them due to the number of hours they spend in front of the screen every day and, specifically, in front of these platforms.

When quarantine was declared due to the Covid-19 pandemic, universities had to take action so that teachers were ready to teach classes through virtual education platforms, the only way to be able to teach classes at that time. Thus, universities in Peru resorted to different strategies to train their teachers. As all the teachers interviewed from private universities told us, the training began immediately, since the universities were concerned about implementing the necessary tools for teaching the courses and that their teachers could handle them correctly as soon as possible, as interviewee number 10 stated. On the other hand, four of the teachers from public universities in Lima and the province did have difficulties in starting classes, with participant 3 stating that "it delayed us, that caused us a lot of pain, a lot of complications, a lot of problems, but we got through it and implemented an "adaptation plan", Like their colleagues in other public universities, they began training months later, starting only in May or June, as interviewees 5 and 7 tell us, that is, two or three months after the regular start of classes, which delayed the start of the cycle during 2020, as in the case of the National University of Ucayali, where classes began only in November, eight months later.

As we were told, all the interviewees received training from their teaching centers to teach their classes using these platforms. Ten of the 10 interviewees continue to receive training on an ongoing basis. Juca (2016: 110) and Cotohuanca (2021: 130) mention that continuous training of teachers is essential to maintain good pedagogy; however, as participant number 6 mentions, at the Universidad Nacional Mayor de

San Marcos, training for teachers was optional, unlike the rest of the universities where it was mandatory from the beginning. In the case of the Universidad Nacional Agraria La Molina, participant number 7 mentions that "there was an intensive training program for teachers at different basic, intermediate and advanced levels for the use of Moodle", but this was done in stages and not all teachers learned at the same time so that the same teachers who already had knowledge in the use of the platforms could train the rest, but for this reason she says that so far they do not feel comfortable using the platform and prefer to use other tools.

Although they all received the corresponding training in their teaching centers, 7 out of 10 perceived that they were not prepared to teach the classes at first, but it was the only way to carry them out and overcome the situation, without paralyzing the classes. As participant number 10 remarks "we depended on the technology", which complements what Viñas (2017: 167) pointed out when referring to the platforms as indispensable tools for the educational process, then it became friendlier and they could handle it with what was necessary to teach their classes. On the contrary, participant number 2 specifies that although this platform could be used for theoretical topics, it could not replace the practical part, because being a pharmacist, her career is experimental and she needed to be in a laboratory to achieve it. Likewise, interviewee number 8 adds that she had to rethink the course and put it together again to be able to dictate it from the virtual education platforms. As commented by 9 of the 10 teachers, in addition to the training provided by the universities themselves, they opted for different techniques complementary to the training and self-training. Participant number 9 mentioned that she practiced and tested within the same platform and investigated by herself the functions and utilities of the platform. Three of the teachers from public universities said that they asked what they did not know to colleagues or family members who know more about the subject. Participant number 4 mentioned that she watched tutorials and referred to the independent search for further training. Participant number 10 also emphasized that she had a technician assigned by the university to support and guide her with the topics related to the platforms.

The case of the two participants from the private universities in the provinces coincides in the use of different mechanisms such as going to a colleague or watching tutorials when they did not have support at the time. Similarly, participant number 2 adds that thanks to the community of her guild she was able to access information and training. There was only one participant, a teacher at a public university in the interior of the country, who mentioned that she was left with only what she received from the training provided by the university itself, i.e., she did without complementary training or self-training. What they all agreed on was that the platforms helped them significantly to keep the course materials more orderly and better organized and that this was beneficial both for them and for the students. Similarly, a comment that came up repeatedly in the interviews was that they would like the platforms to be customized, with specific functions required for each course depending on the needs of each teacher and the areas where they teach.

Challenges faced by teachers and development of competencies during the use of virtual education platforms

For teachers, having to teach their classes through virtual education platforms has meant a radical change, so many of them have encountered challenges during the process and also with the development of new competencies. One of the biggest challenges was the lack of experience in the use of the platforms, although it is true that the teachers of the private universities had more knowledge of these platforms because they had been working with them before; none of them had taught a virtual class until then. Once they finished the training and had to start teaching, an important challenge was to "break their beliefs about technology" as mentioned by participant number 2, to lose their fear and start teaching their classes through the platforms; in the same way, the redesign of the courses was repeated by the teachers because they mentioned that in this process they understood better what was more useful for the teaching of the course. Participant number 3 mentioned that the older teachers at his university "demonized" technology while the rest agreed that it has been a positive change and that they always have to continue exploring and learning new technological tools. Bravo, Rosa; Reynosa, Enaidy; Rivera, Edith and Rodríguez, Darien, (2020: 142) add that teacher training has a close relationship with teachers' mental health. It is here where teachers mention that they have developed technological competence: from the approach of the class to getting to work on it, obtaining a certain mastery of the platform to teach their classes, and finally getting to use new teaching techniques in their activity.

To maintain the interest of the students, they had to calculate their time and use other technological tools such as Jammboard, Kahoot and

Mentimeter, or perhaps place a video that they had previously prepared so that the class takes another direction and the students maintain their interest. All the teachers mentioned that they do not know if their students are really interested or if they are doing other activities at the same time. Since the use of the video camera in on mode is not mandatory, they cannot see the expression of faces and identify who is attentive and who is not, and they recognize that being at home, there are many distracters, including family members, who may interrupt them during class. Likewise, participant number 10 emphasizes that at the beginning the students were more interested in participating, turning on the camera, but nowadays they are bored of being in front of the screen and excuse themselves by saying that they do not have good internet connectivity or that the microphone fails, many with the intention of not turning on the camera or not participating. Similarly, communication skills have been developed. Interviewee 8 mentions that she feels like an announcer, mentioning the following: "the truth is that sometimes I feel like I am on a radio (…) Yes, I have had to develop a new communication skill, to become an announcer". The same interviewee also states that she has always had this communication competence, but that she has only now been able to take advantage of it and feel that it really reaches her students and that they understand her. For this, it is also important that the number of students is adequate, since not being in a conventional classroom makes it difficult to get everyone to participate and feel interested. Two of the interviewees from public universities, one from Lima and the other from the province, mentioned that they have had as many as 100 or 200 students in a class, which has made it difficult for them to know if all the students are really taking advantage of the class, and they mentioned that this should be regulated, and the use of virtuality should not be abused. Another important issue recurrently mentioned by teachers, 4 out of 10 in this case, is the issue of evaluations. Some mention that they have had to adapt the evaluations to be able to make corrections, but an issue that worries them is plagiarism and impersonation, since it is not possible to know for sure if the students deserve the grade they get because they may talk and copy from each other or someone else may do the evaluations for them. Since each one is at home, it is impossible to control this issue or until that moment they could not find a practical solution to it. In this sense, they agree with Cervi, Parola, Tejedor and Tusa (2020: 20) who explain that it is important for teachers that students develop critical and reflective thinking, and this should be reflected in the course. During the entire teaching process, in the preparation of the classes, or uploading content to the platform, as in asynchronous classes, to synchronous classes that are conducted through videoconferencing, teachers recognize that there is a certain relationship between the performance of the class and the medium through which it is taught. Thus, 8 of the 10 affirm that a link is generated with their students, although they also refer to the fact that it does not reach the same level as with face-to-face classes. Only two of the teachers categorically deny having achieved any link with the students because they consider the link through platforms as very distant, this contradicting Anchundia, Arboleda, Astudillo and Pinto (2018: 594) when he points out that the platforms give rise to socialization because they generate a teacher–student approach. But the challenge by which teachers in public universities have been most affected, without excluding those in private universities but to a lesser extent, is that of connectivity, since all interviewees from public universities agree that many of their students live in areas where they do not have good connectivity. Some due to the pandemic had to return to their cities and in the country there are serious connectivity problems, so many of them had to move to places where the internet does reach them or acquire more modern devices. As mentioned by Expósito and Marsollier (2020:18), inequalities were highlighted and made known in terms of access to digital technologies and resources.

When asked: Did you seek individual training to optimize the use of the virtual education platform? The results presented were diverse. Half of the respondents answered that in order to be trained quickly and to be able to use the platforms, they asked a colleague related to computer systems management or someone with more experience than them. The other half was divided between those who sought help from younger family members and those who did seek individual training by exploring the platform or looking for tutorials on YouTube. Only one respondent answered that what they received from the university was enough. It is important to note that this question did not generate a clear division between teachers from private universities and those from public universities. This highlights the importance of independent professional networks in the organization of teaching solutions in the face of Covid-19 and the health emergency.

Conclusions

After analyzing the preparation that teachers had for virtual education platforms during the Covid-19 pandemic, we can conclude that teachers went through different challenges to finally adapt to virtual education and become guides for their students. Those who had no previous experience in the use of virtual education platforms, whether synchronous or asynchronous, had more difficulties in making this adaptation. Teachers had negative perceptions regarding virtual education or new technologies as explained by (Albuquerque, C.; Arteaga, M.; Costas, V.; Muñoz, D.; Porta, M.; Sunday, S.; Tomczyk, Ł.; Yasar, O 2021: 2739) and (Carabelli 2020: 197) when mentioning the different perspectives and experiences of teachers when they were forced to migrate from face-to-face to virtual and take a new direction in their educational agenda.

The teachers confirmed that the virtual education platforms were of great help to organize the content of their courses (Vargas & Villalobos 2018: 23), contributing to the autonomous learning of their students and creating knowledge through them as Gil, Montoya and Sepúlveda (2019: 7) argue. It is important to note that the interviewees mention that the benefits of these platforms can only occur accompanied by a guide directed to the teacher (Vargas & Villalobos, 2018: 22), which also contributes to the dynamism of the class (Barrios, Delgado, Maradey, 2021: 147). Similarly, the use of platforms has been a great advantage in terms of time optimization, since having all the material available in a single digital container influences the immediacy and flexibility of the student's time as mentioned by Carretero and Hermosilla (2004: 142).

Likewise, if they have the appropriate devices and a good Internet connection, they can take their classes without having to travel to their study center, saving time and money in mobilization. Regarding our second specific objective of exploring the competencies acquired by teachers during the use of the platforms, we conclude that there were many challenges that teachers had to face, such as: the late implementation of the platforms, the delay in the start of the trainings and the delay in the school start in public universities, in addition to the State's problems around connectivity. So teachers had to accelerate their media literacy processes (Jooyeun, 2017: 7) so that their students can receive their classes in the best possible way and keep them interested throughout the time that the confinement and virtuality of the classes lasted. It is important to note that resorting to the redesign of their courses, and the use of new technological and communication tools, has improved and developed their media competencies (Lázaro-Cantabrana, Silva & Usart 2019: 34). Similarly, evaluations had to be modified to adapt them to the virtual environment and to a more efficient way of grading (Cabero & Palacios 2021:170).

Focusing on our main objective, focused on analyzing the preparation that higher education teachers had for virtual education through virtual education platforms, we conclude that teachers from private universities had fewer complications because they were accustomed to using these platforms to a large or small extent, thus highlighting the inequalities in the use of technologies and pedagogical resources between private and public systems (Expósito and Marsollier 2020: 19). It is clear that for everyone conducting synchronous classes through videoconferencing was a novelty to which they had to adapt. Most of the interviewees stated that they would like the platforms to be more personalized and have specific functions they need for the courses they teach, without having to be looking for extra tools to the platform. Finally, it should be noted that higher education through virtual education platforms will continue since the pandemic has accelerated the move to virtuality, which does not mean a replacement of face-to-face education, but rather that education should be complementary, teachers propose hybrid education options, currently growing.

This research has sought to help understand the diverse behaviors and different reactions of the Peruvian higher education system with respect to new technologies and how teachers faced difficulties and proposed solutions and strategies in the midst of the Covid-19 pandemic. It is worth mentioning that the research aims to help recognize what aspects can be foreseen and improved within higher education so that teachers find greater access to training in the use of these platforms and mixed teaching methodologies.

We recommend and encourage more geographically specific research, by region, type of universities and type of careers.

Bibliography

Aguaded, Ignacio (2012). "United Nations aiming at media literacy education. UN aiming at media education and media literacy", in *Comunicar*, 38, 7–8.

Agudelo, Mónica (2009). "Importance of instructional design in virtual learning environments", in *New Ideas in Educational Computing*, J. Sánchez (ed.), 5, 118–127.

Albuquerque, C., Arteaga, M., Costas, V., Muñoz, D., Porta, M., Sunday, S., Tomczyk, Ł. and Yasar, O. (2021). "Are teachers techno- optimists or techno-pessimists? A pilot comparative among teachers in Bolivia, Brazil, the Dominican Republic, Ecuador, Finland, Poland, Turkey, and Uruguay", in *Education and Information Technologies*, 26, 2715–2741.

Anchundia, Z. Arboleda, M., Astudillo, M. and Pinto, B. (2018). "Application of ICT as a learning tool in Higher Education", in *RECIMUNDO*, 2 (2), 585–598.

Ara, S.; Magaña, A., Mendoza; E., San Román, K. and Yepez, A. (2019). "Use of educational virtual platforms in university teaching practice – A case study", in *Ibero-American Journal of Science*, 7 (1), 11–19.

Aufderheide, Patricia (1993). *Media Literacy: A Report of the National Leadership Conference on Media Literacy*. Aspen, CO: Aspen Institute.

Barrera, Víctor and Guapi, Ana (2018). "The importance of the use of virtual platforms in higher education" *Revista Atlante,* Education and Development Notebooks, Brazil.

Barrios, L., Delgado, M. and Maradey, J. (2021). "SWOT analysis: educational platforms used by mathematics teachers in Barranquilla – Colombia", in *Recursive Worls Scientific Journal*, 4 (1), 133–148.

Benta, D., Bologa, G. and Dzita, I. (2014). "E-learning Platforms in Higher Education. Case study", in *Procedia Computer Science*, 31, 1170–1173.

Bravo, Rosa, Reynosa, Enaidy, Rivera, Edith and Rodríguez, Darien (2020). "Educational teacher adaptation in the covid-19 context: a systematic review", in *Conrado*, 16 (77), 141–149.

Cabero-Almenara, J. and Palacios-Rodríguez, A. (2021), "The evaluation of virtual education: e-activities", *RIED, Ibero-American Journal of Distance Education,* 24 (2), 169–188.

Cabezas, C., Castro, E., Chowell, G., Cornejo, K., Garro, D., Ibarguen, L., La Torre Rosillo, L., Loayza, M., Mezarina, L., Mimbela, J., Munayco, C., Ordinola, I., Quijano, F., Ramos, W., Reyes, M., Rojas-Vasquez, K., Rothenberg, R., Soto-Cabeza, G., Tariq, A. and Valle, A. (2020). "Early transmission dynamics of COVID-19 in a southern hemisphere setting: Lima-Peru: February 29th -March 30th", in *Infectious Disease Modelling*, 5, 338–345.

Carabelli, Patricia (2020). "Response to the COVID-19 outbreak: Virtual teaching time", *InterChanges, Dilemmas and Transitions in Higher Education*, 7 (2), 189–198.

Carretero M. and Hermosilla, J. (2004). "Knowledge management and generation through the use of digital training platforms", in *Complutense Journal of Education*, 15 (1), 139–164.

Cervi, L; Parola, A.; Tejedor, S. and Tusa, F. (2020). "Education in times of pandemic: reflections of students and teachers on university virtual education in Spain, Italy and Ecuador", in *Latin Journal of Social Communication*, 78, 19–40.

Cisneros-Cohernour, E. J., Cordero Arroyo, G., Espinosa Díaz, Y., García, B., Ponce Ceballos, S., and Serrano, E. L. (2018). "Teaching competencies in virtual environments: a model for their assessment", *RIIbero-American Journal of Distance Education*, 21 (1), 343–365.

Cotohuanca, Sujeidy (2021). "Systematic review: Continuous teacher training on virtual platforms", *Research Journal UPNW*, n. 92, 130–139.

Creswell, J. Ward (2003). *Research design: Qualitative, quantitative, and mixed method approaches*, Thousand Oaks, CA: Sage Publications.

Creswell, J. Ward and Creswell, J. David (2017). *Research design: Qualitative, quantitative, and mixed methods approaches*, Sage Publications.

Expósito, Cristián and Marsollier, Roxana (2020). "Virtuality and education in times of COVID-19. An empiric study in Argentina", *Education and Humanism*, 22 (39), 1–22.

Ferrés, Joan and Piscitelli, Alejandro (2012). "Media competence. Articulated proposal of dimensions and indicators", *Comunicar*, 38, 75–82.

Flick, Uwe (2015). *The Qualitative Research Design*. Madrid: Morata.

Gastelo, Rosy, Maguiña, Ciro and Tequen, Arly (2020). "The new Coronavirus and the Covid-19 pandemic", in *Herediana Medical Journal*, 31(2), 125–131.

Gil, V.; Montoya, L. and Sepúlveda, J. (2019). "Role of virtual educational platforms in engineering education", *EIEI ACOFI*, 2 (1), 1–9.

González-Monteagudo, José (2001). "The interpretative paradigm in social and educational research: New answers to old questions ", Cuestiones pedagógicas, 15, Universidad de Sevilla, pp. 227–240.

Hernández, L., Loor, T., Palma, A. and Salazar, G. (2021), "Technology: impact on the synchronous and asynchronous teaching-learning process in the public universities of Manabí", in *Atlante Journal: Education and Development Notebooks*, 13 (5), 97–116.

Herrera, M., Pinto, D., Valdivia, A., (2018), "Media literacy and learning. Conceptual contribution in the field of communication-education", in *Educare Electronic Journal*, 22 (2), 1–16.

Jooyeun, P (2017), "Media literacy, media competence and media policy in the digital age", *Hawaii University International Conferences*, 1–12.

Juca, Fernando (2016), "Distance education, a necessity for the training of professionals", *University and Society Journal*, 8 (1), 106–111.

Kvale Steinar (2011). "Interviews in qualitative research", Madrid: Morata.

Lázaro-Cantabrana, J. Silva, J. and Usart, M. (2019). "Teacher's digital competence among final year pedagogy students in Chile and Uruguay",in *Comunicar*, 61, 33–43.

López, Gabriel (2020). "New challenges of virtual education, immersive simulation as a future for education", *CEMA Working Papers: Working Papers Series*, 769, 1–19.

Miyahira, Juan (2020). "What the pandemic can bring us", in *Herediana Medical Journal*, 31 (2), 83–84.

Palma, J., Romero, W., Soledispa, C. and Zuña, E. (2020). "Virtual platforms and promotion of collaborative learning in high education students", in *Educational Synergies*, 1 (5), 349–369.

Potter, James (2010), "The state of media literacy", in *Journal of Broadcasting & Electronic Media*, 54 (4), 675–696.

United Nations Educational, Scientific and Cultural Organization, (2020). "Media and Information Literacy in the Age of Uncertainty".

United Nations Educational, Scientific and Cultural Organization (2021). "UNESCO's Response to COVID-19".

Vargas-Jiménez, I. (2012). "The interview in the qualitative research: trends and challengers", in *Electronic Journal Quality In Higher Education*, 3 (1), 119–139.

Vargas, A. & Villalobos, G. (2018). "The use of virtual platforms and their impact on the learning process in the subjects of Criminology and Police Science majors at the Universidad Estatal a Distancia de Costa Rica". In *Educare Electronic Magazine*, 22 (1), 20–39.

Viñas, M (2017). "The importance of the use of educational platforms", in *Letras Journal*, 1 (6), 157–169.

Wang, K. Zhang, Q. and Zhou, S, (2020). "Application and practice of VR virtual education platform in improving the quality and ability of college students", in *IEEE Access*, 8, 162830–162837.

World Health Organization, (2021), "Background information on COVID-19", https://apps.who.int/iris/bitstream/handle/10665/332197/WHO-2019-nCoV-FAQ-Virus_origin-2020.1-eng.pdf

The July 11, 2021, protests in Cuba: A unique event?

ORLANDO MANZANO GUERRERO. *Recherches sur les Suds et les Orients, UR4582.*
Montpellier 3

Introduction

In the concert of Latin American and Caribbean nations, with which it shares a common geography and a large part of its history, Cuba stands out for having certain peculiarities that make it a unique case. Its historical trajectory throughout the 20th century – and, in particular, the political, economic and social path it has taken since the triumph of its Revolution in 1959 – has got clearly much to do with this. Social protest, a topic in which the region has overall a long tradition, is today one of the main areas in which the island differs from its neighbours. The difficulties faced by its ailing economy and the repercussions it has had on its population are often subjects for discussion; incidents of civil unrest or political instability in the country are much rarer. That is why the images that went around the world on July 11, 2021,[1] showing thousands of people demonstrating in the streets of several Cuban cities, were at first so particularly striking. These images were all the more remarkable, considering they came at a time when the lives of the island's inhabitants – like those of the rest of the world – seemed to be at a standstill, after several months of crisis resulting from the Covid-19 pandemic.

Within this framework, the aim of this chapter is to analyse the specific circumstances in which the 11J protests took place in Cuba, in order to elucidate to what extent they constitute a unique event. To do so, we

---

[1] In the following days some protests – isolated and of lesser intensity – were also reported in various locations throughout the country. In the absence of sufficient information on these, we focus here on the events that took place on July 11. For the sake of simplicity, we refer to this date in our text as 11J.

will first try to determine as objectively as possible what happened that day and why. We will then put the events in perspective, both geographically and historically, to shed light on some of their main peculiarities. Finally, we will frame these events in the global context in which they occurred, with a view to clarifying how they relate to the social dynamics witnessed at the time in various parts of the world.

Understanding the keys to 11J

Any analysis of the events of 11J requires, first and foremost, establishing as impartially and objectively as possible what really happened on that day, as well as the reasons that may have led to it. However, it must be acknowledged that this is not an easy task, due to the differing versions and interpretations of those events given at the time by detractors and supporters of the Cuban political regime, both inside and outside the country. In parallel with the events, a constant flow of news, videos and photos were disseminated through social networks and the media, showing diverse, or even opposing, perspectives of what was happening on the streets of Cuba. The war of images that ensued made it difficult to distinguish where information ended and misinformation began, leading to often incomplete or erroneous conclusions about the events.

The images that circulated outside the island showed crowds of mainly young people, demonstrating in several Cuban cities – generally peacefully – and shouting "we want freedom", "down with the dictatorship", "democracy is respect", "we are not afraid", among many other slogans of political and social content. According to foreign correspondents accredited in Cuba,[2] the first outbursts took place in a small town southwest of the capital. Reportedly, dozens of inhabitants took to the streets there in order to protest against food and medicine shortages, as well as the government's insufficient response to the resurgent Covid-19 pandemic. Clashes with security forces in different parts of the country were also shown during the course of the day, as well as the arrest of dozens of protesters who were seen being quickly removed from the scene in police vehicles. These images were presented to the world as irrefutable evidence of what was interpreted as a massive popular uprising in favour

---

[2] Read, for example: Vicent, Mauricio, "Cuba vive las mayores protestas contra el Gobierno desde la crisis de los años noventa", *El País*, July 12, 2021.

of structural changes in the island's political system; an uprising that did not achieve its objectives due to the police brutality with which it was repressed, the intransigence of the main leaders of the communist party and the national government, and the severity with which the courts later judged those who were arrested that day.[3]

For some Latin American academics, it was nevertheless a decisive milestone in the history of the Caribbean nation, which has already become installed in the collective imagination to the point of marking "a before and after". Writer Mario Vargas Llosa considered it nothing less than "the beginning of the end" of the "Castro regime".[4] Political scientist and historian Armando Chaguaceda shared a similar opinion. For him, the beginning of a new era was possible after what he defined as a true "social explosion" that managed to alter "profoundly the balance of power prevailing until then, between the communist regime and the population". From now on, he argued, "it will be difficult to consider the island as a static society living under the yoke of a power that has made a deliberate decision to distance itself from its people, who is driven by a desire for freedom".[5] According to this view, the events of 11J were thus an important turning point with potential repercussions for the future of the Cuban people.

The account of those events and the conclusions drawn from them by the island's media[6] differed markedly from the above. To begin with, they stressed the illegal nature of what was labelled from the outset as "riots" and "acts of vandalism" that disturbed the usual peace and quiet of the people. The actions of "disruptive individuals" who sought only to damage socialist state property and attack those who think differently were denounced. To support such allegations, images were shown of people overturning police cars in the street, assaulting law enforcement officers and looting shops selling food and household appliances.[7] Soon,

---

[3] Multiple examples of testimonies, articles and links confirming this version of events are available on the website https://cubajulio11.com/.
[4] Vargas Llosa, Mario, "El principio del fin", *El País*, July 25, 2021.
[5] Chaguaceda, Armando, and Melissa Cordero Novo, "Estallido social en Cuba. El fin de la épica redentora", *Le Grand Continent*, July 23, 2021.
[6] Cuban television, radio and print media are all state-owned and offer little or no scope for the presentation of views different from the official government version.
[7] See, for example, the TV report "Cuba: ¿Qué ocurrió en Cárdenas el 11 de julio?", posted on *Canal Caribe's* YouTube channel on July 15, 2021.

it all gave way to other images in which mass marches involving even local or national government leaders could be witnessed. Using the same kind of mobile devices as those who shared anti-government protests on social media around the world, thousands of people were filmed carrying Cuban flags, banners and pictures of current and historical political leaders; shouting slogans in favour of the government and against the United States – which they blamed for inciting a social explosion by causing the food shortages and electricity supply problems that the Cuban population was then facing.

Incidentally, in the media coverage and multiple television appearances by Cuban President Miguel Díaz-Canel during and after the events, mention was made of a small number of peaceful demonstrators who might have felt genuinely exhausted by the shortages and irregular energy supply, as well as by the pandemic fatigue in the midst of the most critical period of Covid-19 in the country. However, the vast majority of those who took to the streets that day were described as "scum", "counter-revolutionaries" and "delinquents". Calls were thus made for "the people [...] to defend the revolution (and) their rights" in the face of "provocations" allegedly promoted by US-funded opposition groups.[8] Therefore, by focusing almost exclusively on acts of violence and degradation of public property – which were indeed committed – and on the strong reaction of disapproval of such acts by the majority of the population, the protests in favour of changes in the current socialist model – which also took place – were made less visible. At the same time, by accusing the US authorities of carrying out "a policy of economic asphyxiation" and "a political-communication campaign" against Cuba, with the aim of generating "misunderstandings and dissatisfaction" among the population, the national leadership would be exonerated in the eyes of the public of any responsibility for the events of 11J or for the poor socio-economic conditions that might have motivated them.

Such conclusions were widely shared by the academic community on the island. Thus, for example, for Frank Josué Solar Cabrales, PhD in Historical Sciences (Solar Cabrales 2021: 12–13), although some citizens

---

[8] Read the article commenting on and analysing the Cuban president's address on television, published in the official newspaper of the Communist Party of Cuba: Ramos López, Gladys Leidys, "A la Revolución la defendemos ante todo", *Granma*, July 12, 2021.

"with legitimate claims and demands" may have joined the demonstrations, these were mostly made of "violent and loutish acts"; a far cry from the narrative promoted abroad. According to him, the riots of that day would have been nothing more than "the materialisation of a strategy of subversion and destabilisation, orchestrated, designed and financed from abroad, with the declared purpose of overthrowing the Cuban Revolution. […] a well thought out manoeuvre (that) forms part of the unconventional war waged for months against Cuba, after stepping up pressure to create material shortages, especially of medicines, food and fuel, with the aim of promoting a social explosion". The failure of this manoeuvre, Solar Cabrales stressed, was mainly due to its limited ability to mobilize the popular sectors at which it was aimed. It was therefore false to claim that the events of 11J had occurred spontaneously, and illusory to expect that they could bring about any change in the country in the short, medium or long term.

These interpretations reflected very different views of the events, their motives and even their possible consequences. If we simply look at the facts, we must acknowledge that the protests, looting and riots that took place across the island of Cuba were indeed intense – even violent – but they were rather brief and did not have widespread popular support. Consider that most of these events took place during the afternoon of July 11 and – according to the most optimistic estimates, the accuracy of which is difficult to prove – some 15,000 people took part in them.[9] In proportion to the number of inhabitants in the country: 11,113,215 people at the end of 2021 (Oficina Nacional de Estadísticas e Información 2022), such figures represented about 0.13 % of the population. On the other hand, it is clear that broad sectors of civil society disapproved of what happened that day. The images of numerous Cubans responding favourably to the authorities' call to "defend the homeland" effectively showed the considerable support that the government still enjoys.

Such images may also have had a dissuasive effect on those who hesitated to join the protests, which may partly explain their rather short-lived nature and the relative low turnout. Other reasons that undoubtedly played a role were the strong reaction of the country's political leadership and security forces, the swift judicial response, and the harsh sentences that resulted from it. In this regard, it is worth noting that in the first

---

[9] According to estimates published on the website https://cubajulio11.com/.

trials that began shortly after the events dozens of demonstrators were brought before the courts on charges of public disorder, incitement to commit a crime or contempt of court – offences punishable by up to one year in prison under the Cuban Penal Code. Trials for violent acts, looting of shops and clashes with police took longer and came up with much more severe convictions: on March 16, 2022, Cuba's Supreme People's Court announced 128 sentences of up to 30 years' imprisonment for these offences. Although it was assured that such convictions were in accordance with the country's legal norms and that no demonstrator had been convicted for political reasons,[10] the truth is that for a large part of the international community these sentences were "excessive" and "disproportionate". Josep Borrel – the European Union's High Representative for Foreign Policy – expressed himself in these terms in a statement in which he called on the island's authorities to respect "the civil and political rights of Cubans, including freedom of association, freedom of assembly and freedom of expression".[11]

On the other hand, the 11J protestors expressed numerous, clear and unambiguous demands for regime change in Cuba. The actions – whether peaceful or violent – of the vast majority of people who took to the streets that day were nonetheless essentially motivated by the scarcity of food, medicines and basic necessities, as well as by the irregularity of the energy supply and the strict health measures imposed on the population since the beginning of the pandemic. Rather than a well-planned, coordinated and targeted collective action, all this points to a desperate reaction by several thousand citizens to the critical socio-economic and health situation prevailing at the time, and to the dissatisfaction of many of them with the way the island's political leaders were handling such situation.

It is not fortuitous that this reaction and the growing popular discontent it reflected should have taken place in a country that has been plagued for several years now by an acute economic crisis whose consequences for the well-being and quality of life of its population have been dire.[12] Some of the

---

[10] See: Torres Corona, Michel E., "¿Presos políticos en Cuba?", *Granma*, February 5, 2022.

[11] Statement included in a press release: "Cuba: Declaración del Alto Representante en nombre de la Unión Europea sobre los juicios y sentencias relativos a las manifestaciones del 11 y 12 de julio de 2021", *European Council*, March 30, 2022.

[12] For a detailed analysis of the setback experienced by Cuba's macroeconomic and social indicators in recent years, see: Mesa-Lago, Carmelo (2021), "Las causas de las protestas y la magnitud de la crisis económica en Cuba", in *Horizonte Cubano*.

main demands that were heard that day, and even the fact that shops selling food and basic necessities were looted, are proof of the importance of the economic factor among the triggers of the events studied here. For most observers of the Cuban reality, the claims put forward by the country's political authorities blaming the poor situation on the embargo imposed by the United States are not entirely unfounded; especially after the application of strong economic sanctions by the Donald Trump administration, reversing the process of rapprochement initiated by President Barack Obama shortly before leaving office. That being said, as Carmelo Mesa-Lago (Mesa-Lago 2021) – a Cuban-born professor whose opinions are a reference on economic issues – stresses, the crisis has in fact multiple causes. Among others, Mesa-Lago points to the economic collapse of Venezuela, the island's main political ally and oil supplier; the Cuban economy's own structural deficiencies; the drastic drop in domestic production that prevented Cuba from fully financing imports with its own exports; erroneous decisions taken at the beginning of 2021 by the Cuban government on economic policy issues, which implied an increase in salaries and pensions but at the same time pushed up prices; the recent process of monetary unification carried out in the country that led to the dollarization of the economy; and so on. All these factors – structural and cyclical, exogenous and endogenous – were therefore responsible to a greater or lesser degree for the severe hardship that Cubans had to endure at the time.

To the above must of course be added the extremely adverse effects of the Covid-19 pandemic, not only in the economic sphere but also from health and social perspectives. First of all, it is clear that the sharp fall in Cuban GDP in 2020 (-10.9 %, one of the largest annual variations in Latin America and the Caribbean) and its almost zero growth (+ 0.5 %) projected for 2021 (ECLAC 2022a: 138),[13] resulted in large part from the situation created by the coronavirus. On the one hand, the extraordinary measures implemented by the national authorities to contain its spread led, among other things, to almost total paralysis of multiple activities related to international tourism – one of the main sources of foreign currency earnings for the Cuban economy. According to Mesa-Lago (2021), "gross income from tourism […] in 2020 fell 80 % compared to 2017". In 2021, revenues were likely to be much lower, given that the number

---

[13] The Economic Commission for Latin America and the Caribbean, known as ECLAC (or CEPAL in Spanish), is a United Nations regional commission to encourage economic cooperation.

of international visitors was also lower: 356,470, or 32.8 % of the 2020 total (ONEI 2021). On the other hand, the slump in international trade deprived the country of much-needed export revenues – down 12.2 % in 2021 from the previous year[14] – and of key imported resources on which its people vitally depend; such as crude oil, food and many other commodities.

In terms of public health, the damage was also severe despite the remarkable progress made by the island in this area. First and foremost, Cuba is now one of the few countries in the world that has managed to produce several Covid-19 vaccines. In August 2020, it became the first country in the region to authorize clinical trials of a candidate vaccine – *Soberana 01* – and then went on to develop four others: *Soberana 02, Abdala, Mambisa* and *Soberana Plus*. Initially, the measures implemented also enabled the government to effectively control the spread of the virus, considerably limiting the number of infections and deaths by 2020: of the 112,441 deaths reported on the island for that year, only 143 were attributed to Covid-19.[15] In 2021, however, the health situation on the national territory became particularly complex, especially around the time of the 11J protests. This was mainly due to the spread of variants with higher transmissibility and severity of infections at a time when mass vaccination of the population had not yet started.[16] It was not until July 9 that the *Centro para el Control Estatal de Medicamentos, Equipos y Dispositivos Médicos* (Centre for State Control of Medicines, Equipment and Medical Devices) – the Cuban regulatory authority – authorized the emergency use of the first of five vaccine candidates developed on the island. This decision came at the time of the worst outbreak of the epidemic up to that moment, with thousands of daily cases of infection and hospital admissions, as well as dozens of deaths, even among people in age groups initially considered to be at low risk. For example, that year the number of deaths due to Covid-19 in people under 60 years of age

---

[14] Source: Cuba. Exportaciones de Mercancías, *Expansión, datosmacro.com*, 2022.

[15] The number of infections was also very limited: 12,056 cases reported, for a rate of 107.6 cases per 100,000 people. Source: Dirección de Registros Médicos y Estadísticas de Salud del Ministerio de Salud Pública de Cuba (2021), *Anuario Estadístico de Salud 2020*, 11–13.

[16] By the end of 2021, however, the situation had improved substantially: 85.5 % of the Cuban population had being fully vaccinated, well above the average for countries in the region. Source: ECLAC (2022b), *Panorama Social de América Latina, 2021*, Santiago de Chile, 110.

"more than doubled" the rates reported for 2020 (ECLAC 2022b: 19). Finally, the collapse of medical care services in several Cuban municipalities and provinces would be an additional, albeit unnecessary, sign of the serious epidemiological situation the country was going through at the time.

But the challenges faced by the island's inhabitants went beyond infection or death from the coronavirus and also affected their living conditions. Access to medicines and health care, employment, and even basic foodstuffs and necessities was also severely limited as a result of the situation created by the pandemic. At the same time, power outages – due to power plant breakdowns and fuel shortages in the country – became longer and more frequent. It was the accumulation of all these social, health and economic problems, which contributed to exacerbating the crisis that had been dragging on for some time and whose solution did not seem to be really within the reach of the national political leadership, that finally provoked – beyond the existence or not of a destabilizing plan encouraged from outside the island – the state of despair that led several thousand people to participate in the protests and riots of 11J. All things considered that these events took place precisely in such a complex and uncertain context is not really surprising.

The peculiarities of 11J

Once the events and their main triggers have been clarified, it would be appropriate to analyse them from a broader perspective, both geographically and historically, in order to shed light on some aspects that allow us to stress their atypical and singular nature. As stated above, the incidents of 11J were characterized first and foremost by their relative short duration and the fact that they enjoyed rather limited popular support. Likewise, it was noted that these incidents were largely motivated by the lack of food and other basic products, as well as by the serious economic and health situation faced at the time by the Cuban population as a whole. This contrasts sharply with what was observed in other situations of civil conflict and/or political unrest witnessed in specific parts of Latin America around the same time. There were indeed several cases of protest demonstrations – some organized, others more spontaneous – that gradually turned into genuine social outbursts which, in addition to their extraordinary duration and geographical spread, had in common the fact that they gave way to a broad convergence of demands by numerous social sectors – thus exposing multiple causes of citizen unrest. Let us briefly look at two of the most notable examples in this regard.

Colombia is one of the settings where the most far-reaching events have taken place, after the first wave of demonstrations which lasted from November 21, 2019, to February 21, 2020. It was a national protest led by trade unions, students, indigenous people, teachers and opposition political sectors that sought mainly to obtain improvements in state social services and employment. Although the marches had to be stopped due to the health emergency crisis caused by the Covid-19 pandemic, popular discontent with the policies of Iván Duque's government did not cease; it became evident again in 2021 after the president's continuous attempts to implement economic measures that would mainly affect the middle class.[17] Although the government eventually withdrew its reform proposal, the demonstrations – whose second wave began on April 28 – continued throughout the year, now focusing on denouncing the disproportionate use of force by members of the police, as well as on renewing the demands for improvements in the social sphere. Equally massive and extensive were the protests that originated in Santiago de Chile and then spread to various cities in the Andean country. These protests, which essentially took place between October 2019 and March 2020, also mobilized several million people. The trigger in this case was the increase in public transport fares in the Chilean capital. Thousands of high school students organized not to pay for the city's Metro and the situation escalated with the multiplication of incidents at underground railway stations and clashes between the crowds and the *carabineros*.[18] Although the Chilean government finally decided not to implement the fare hike, new hotbeds of conflict soon appeared in other regions exposing deeper reasons for frustration – such as inequality and the precariousness of the middle and lower classes, or the rejection of the political class and state institutions.[19]

---

[17] On the motives, development and impact of the Colombian protests, see: International Crisis Group, "Paro y pandemia: las respuestas a las protestas masivas en Colombia", *Latin America Report*, 90, July 2, 2021.

[18] The Chilean police.

[19] See an analysis of these protests by Chilean political scientist Rossana Castiglioni at the debate on democracy and social protest in Latin America, organized by the *Latin American Studies Association* on May 28, 2021.

In both cases – like in several others that took place almost simultaneously throughout Latin America – the extraordinary level of intensity, transversality and extension in time and space reached by the protest demonstrations is noteworthy. They clearly form part of the type of social movements that Jorge Alonso Sánchez (Alonso Sánchez 2020: 24–25) describes as "multi-class and multi-sectoral". As the renowned Mexican researcher and academic points out, these are movements from which "a wide range of demands emerge that fundamentally question the prevailing order" and whose genesis and evolution are, in general, the following:

> ... small movements that are resisting exploitation, oppression and domination, nurture larger mobilisations, because when intolerable situations break out, it quickly sparks off these movements, as well as other groups that were not previously involved but share common concerns. This leads to large movements that manage to reach more people and arouse indignation. At times of mass decline, the former movements return to their resistance, but with the lessons learned from the larger movement. There are new nuclei that remain as active as the smaller groups, and their impact depends on the converging views that are generated. It should not be forgotten that mobilisation cannot be continuous or linear; that there are setbacks and defeats, so that mobilisations seem to disappear, but nuclei of active minorities and other expressions of multiple resistances remain.

It is clear that such a description should in no way be applied to the events that took place in Cuba. Even though these events effectively revealed a situation with which the vast majority of the island's population could have identified, they did not manage to go beyond what – to a certain extent – resembles the first stage defined by Alonso Sánchez.

Another striking aspect of the events of 11J was the perceived violence during the riots and acts of vandalism on which the national press and authorities focused their attention, as well as the clashes with law enforcement that took place in the context, or on the fringes, of the protests. Such violence resulted not only in dozens of injuries and the arrest, prosecution and sentencing of more than a hundred people but also in the death of at least one individual at the hands of a Cuban police officer.[20]

---

[20] As acknowledged by the Cuban Ministry of the Interior (MININT) in a press release published on the website of *Radio Rebelde*, later reproduced by other national media, the death of one of the participants in the riots occurred on the afternoon of July 12 during a confrontation with law enforcement officers. Although the MININT stated that it regretted "the death of this person, [...] in the midst of a complex scenario in

Without wishing to downplay the seriousness of these events, it must be acknowledged that they were on a much smaller scale than what was seen in other parts of the region, where the greater degree of radicalism and aggressiveness of the popular uprisings was consubstantial with the extreme harshness of the repression unleashed by the national authorities in an attempt to put an end to them.

The two cases mentioned above are once again paradigmatic examples in this regard. Both the Colombian and Chilean governments declared multiple states of emergency, night-time curfews and even the deployment of the army in major cities. These measures sought to curb the violence unleashed on the streets in parallel to the marches, sit-ins, road blockades and *cacerolazos*[21] that – in a non-consecutive manner – took place throughout the period. As a result, in both cases the number of injured, detained, disappeared and dead was surprisingly high. A report published in June 2021 by Human Rights Watch[22] documented, for example, the use of live ammunition by the Colombian police, resulting in at least 16 deaths in the country. The same report denounced the arbitrary dispersal of rallies through the use of non-lethal weapons such as tear gas, beatings of demonstrators and even sexual abuse of some of them. For its part, the Colombian Ministry of Defence reported[23] the death of two officers and more than 1450 injured as a result of attacks directed against the security forces. Alonso Sánchez (2020: 38) also echoes several reports of serious human rights violations by the Chilean state, including "412 cases of torture, 191 cases of sexual violence, 3,649 injured people, (including) 405 cases of eye injuries" following the use of non-lethal weapons by the

---

which public peace and order is being preserved", the exact circumstances in which it occurred and the name of the policeman involved in the events were not known until later. According to reports, the Cuban Public Prosecutor's Office had exonerated the latter of charges on the grounds of "self-defence"; a version considered unlikely and a decision questioned by media and human rights organizations based abroad. For more details, read: "Nota Informativa sobre el fallecimiento de un ciudadano cubano", *Radio Rebelde*, July 13, 2022 and "¿Qué pasó en La Güinera el 11 de julio? Exigen investigación independiente sobre muerte de manifestante", *Radio Televisión Martí*, August 14, 2021.

[21] A form of popular protest practised in certain Spanish-speaking countries, which consists in a group of people creating noise by banging pots, pans and other utensils in order to call for attention.

[22] "Colombia: Egregious Police Abuses Against Protesters", *Human Rights Watch*, June 9, 2021.

[23] "Balance General - Paro Nacional", *Colombian Ministry of Defence*, June 25, 2021.

anti-riot forces. This was by no means exclusive of the events discussed here; it was one of the main common features shared by many of the social outbursts[24] that shook countries in the region around the time the events of 11J took place in Cuba. The particularity of the latter lies precisely in the less radical and less violent nature they fortunately had.

Finally, it was pointed out that contrary to what many demonstrators and foreign observers expected – and unless there is a radical change in the near future that disproves this assertion – 11J in no way brought about "the beginning of the end" of the "Castro regime". Here is another significant difference with some of the most symbolic cases of Latin American social movements which have had considerable direct repercussions for the lives of the people. Such is the case again with Chile. As a result of the massive demonstrations there, the then president Sebastián Piñera was forced to announce several bills and reforms aimed at addressing some of the protesters' main demands.[25] In addition, an agreement signed on November 15, 2019, between the government and the majority of parties represented in Congress gave the green light to the convening of a historic national plebiscite that would lead to the drafting and subsequent approval of a new Constitution and, later, to the victory of left-wing presidential candidate Gabriel Boric in the December 2021 elections. What happened in Bolivia in November 2019 – albeit with many specificities of its own – bears similarities to the previous example, in that what began as a social outburst against the government in power ultimately led to a change of political regime. In this case, however, the divorce between the authorities and part of the popular movement occurred in the midst of a

---

[24] Another example is Venezuela; a country with one of the highest rates of social and political conflicts on the continent which, with a total of 16,739 demonstrations (some 46 per day) in 2019 broke the record number of protests recorded there in the last nine years (Observatorio Venezolano de Conflictividad Social: 2020). All this in the midst of a serious political and institutional crisis whose climax was the decision taken within the National Assembly to declare that Nicolás Maduro was "usurping" his office, following which Juan Guaidó – as president of the Assembly – was sworn in as interim president of the Republic in January 2019. From then on, demonstrations for and against the Maduro government, riots, looting and repression were almost constant until the end of the year and – as in Colombia and Chile – resulted in several dozen deaths, injuries and hundreds of arrests.

[25] On the measures communicated, see: "Presidente Piñera anuncia Agenda Social con mayores pensiones, aumento del ingreso mínimo, freno al costo de la electricidad, beneficios en salud, nuevos impuestos para altas rentas y defensoría para víctimas de delitos", *Presidencia de la República*, October 23, 2019.

social and political crisis triggered by allegations of fraud in the October 20 presidential elections. This led President Evo Morales – in power for almost 14 years – to resign from office and leave his country,[26] after which right-wing opposition leader Jeanine Áñez declared herself interim president of the Bolivian government. Unlike these examples of social movements that were at the origin of a profound process that questioned the *status quo* in their respective countries, the Cuban protests did not – at least in the short term – have any major political or social implications.

In short, the social conflicts mentioned here – despite their different origins, ideological lines and outcomes – have in common the extraordinary level of intensity, transversality and extension in time and space that they achieved. Particularly striking was also the extreme violence of the riots and clashes that took place in parallel to the protest demonstrations. In some cases, the social and political advances they brought about were also significant. It is clear from such examples that the events of 11J have to be seen on a much smaller scale, which is what fundamentally defines their atypical nature. Contrary to what was observed in several Latin American countries, the events on the Caribbean island did not have the impact and scope that would have justified labelling them as a social explosion.

That being said, it would be a mistake to minimize the relevance of these events. A quick glance at the country's history since the triumph of its Revolution in 1959 does indeed reveal the extraordinary nature of the events under study. Traditionally, when Cubans mobilize, they do so to pay homage to a patriotic hero, to demonstrate their support for the government and its leaders and/or to express their rejection of what is described on the island as "attacks by US imperialism" and its accomplices aimed at "destroying the social and political gains of the Revolution". These mass marches take place periodically – on important dates – or occasionally, but always after being called by mass organizations,[27] the

---

[26] It is worth noting that for some scholars, including Jorge Alonso Sánchez (2020: 32), Morales did not actually resign from office but was overthrown by a coup d'état. In any case, as the same author points out, the social organizations did not support the left-wing leader at decisive moments, and all the military (authors of the supposed coup) had to do was to play their cards once the government had been overcome by reaction in the streets.

[27] Mass organizations were created or reorganized after the triumph of the Revolution and generally function as structures of social control and mobilization. Among the most influential are the *Central de Trabajadores de Cuba* (the country's only legally

Communist Party or the government itself. They generally conclude with events during which political leaders or representatives of these organizations make speeches and appeal for the support of the population. What is really unusual is to see mobilizations, whether peaceful or violent, in which thousands of people go out to openly and massively protest against the actions of the national leadership, or even to show their discontent with the economic situation of the country. That this happened on 11J took everyone by surprise, including the government, citizens and outside observers. As political scientist Javier Corrales points out, "in the past, protests were limited to tiny groups, especially in Havana, the capital. Ordinary Cubans, even non-conformists, knew not to get too close to the protesters, either physically or politically. Any expression of solidarity with any form of dissent is quite risky. Losing your job is common, as is being arrested".[28]

On the one hand, it is true that over the last six decades there have been few protests in Cuba and these have always been extremely limited in terms of the number of participants and the territorial extension they have achieved. The most important one took place on August 5, 1994 in front of the *Malecón*, Havana's well-known seafront promenade. On that day, hundreds of the capital's inhabitants gathered there to complain about the serious economic crisis they were experiencing at the time and to call their leaders to account. That episode is best remembered for the fact that it triggered one of the largest waves of migration to the United States in the country's recent history. It was the so-called "Rafting Crisis",[29] during which over 30,000 Cubans reportedly left the island. The scope of the protest as such was otherwise quite limited. The weak popular support it received, together with the presence on the streets of Havana of the leader of the Revolution, Fidel Castro Ruz, and the rapid

---

constituted trade union), the Federation of University Students, the Federation of Cuban Women and the Committees for the Defence of the Revolution. On this subject, see: Marie Laure Geoffray (2012), *Contester à Cuba*, Paris, Editions Dalloz, 2012, 2.

[28] Corrales, Javier, "El día en que los cubanos perdieron el miedo", *The New York Times*, July 14, 2021.

[29] For more information on this subject, see the paper presented by Siro del Castillo at the symposium "Recordando la crisis de los balseros y sus consecuencias, 20 años después", sponsored by the Cuban Research Institute of Florida International University, on September 4, 2014.

intervention of the forces of law and order and civilians sympathetic to the government, helped to put an end to it in just a few hours.

Not even the wave of citizen protests that began in 2011 in various parts of the world, giving rise to what has been called "the most revolutionary era in history"[30] had any impact on the Caribbean island. These popular revolts, initiated by the Arab Spring, the Spanish 15M and Occupy Wall Street in the United States, were characterized – as evoked in a study published by Oxfam International (Oxfam International 2016: 5–13) – by their "heterogeneous, polysemic and polyclassist" nature. They were composed of "connected crowds and circumstantial actors" and marked a turning point in terms of the format and flow of social demonstrations on a global scale, "both in democratic countries and in those ruled by authoritarian regimes". Cuba, contrary to what happened in many Latin American countries, once again remained on the sidelines of such events.

This does not mean, of course, that there has never been any form of protest there. The French political scientist Marie Laure Geoffray (Geoffray 2012: 2–3) has, for example, documented the existence since the mid-1990s of different groups that share objectives of social change and adopt "similar unconventional practices of protest, through the creation of a hybrid repertoire at the intersection of cultural creation and collective action". Likewise, for several decades now, individual expressions of despair and criticism of the country's socio-economic situation have become increasingly frequent and widespread. These groups or individual expressions of discontent have, however, lacked sufficient force to give rise to large-scale protest mobilizations or collective and organized demands against the regime. The increase in the number of political dissidents, which is difficult to quantify, is part of the same dynamic. There is indeed an internal dissidence movement – which has been growing since the 1990s – whose main objective has always been to push for a transition to democracy on the island. However, its reach and impact on Cuban civil society have historically been very limited.

On the other hand, it is also true that dissent, freedom of demonstration or association are hardly tolerated on the island. As Cuban jurist

---

[30] This expression is used in the study "Nuevas dinámicas de comunicación, organización y acción social en América Latina. Reconfiguraciones tecnopolíticas", *Oxfam international*, 2016, 3.

José A. García Veloso[31] emphasizes, the Constitution of the Republic of Cuba recognizes freedom of expression as a right of all citizens. He cites as proof Article 54, which stipulates: "The State recognises, respects and guarantees people's freedom of thought, conscience and expression". He also points out that the Penal Code currently in force protects this right in Article 291: "'Crime against the free expression of thought' is the name of the rule, which prohibits and punishes preventing others, in any way, from exercising the right to freedom of speech or press guaranteed by the Constitution and the laws; with a modality that provides for a higher penalty when the crime is committed by a public official, with abuse of his position". It should be noted, however, that in practice, the expression of anti-government ideas – especially in public spaces – can be punishable by prison sentences. If it is considered as an incitement "against the social order, [...] or the socialist state", this type of demonstration can effectively be equated with "enemy propaganda", in which case it is "punishable by imprisonment for one to eight years".[32] This explains to a large extent the almost total absence of citizen protests in favour of social and political change in Cuba. It is not, of course, the only reason.

During the first decades of the Revolution, people's adherence to government policies – and therefore, the absence of social protest – was mainly due to the progress it brought about in terms of social justice and equality and access to housing, health and education. That progress was framed, not without reason, as far superior to the standards of other countries and in particular those of regional neighbours. Over time, Cuba began to experience long periods of economic crisis, especially after the downfall of the socialist bloc in the early 1990s. This caused hardship and an increase in the cost of living with dire effects for the majority of the population. Yet, it did not encourage the search for an alternative social project through protest. For the French researcher Vincent Bloch (Bloch 2009: 83–104), this situation was partly the result of a process of adaptation on the part of Cubans; the hope of improving their financial situation, a priority shared by the vast majority of them, was in fact consubstantial with a slowing down of criticism of the political order

---

[31] García Veloso, José A., "La libertad de expression", *La Joven Cuba*, November 25, 2020.
[32] According to Article 103.1 of the Penal Code of December 29, 1989, *Gaceta Oficial de la República de Cuba*.

in force in the country.³³ To cope with the shortage of basic consumer goods, large sectors of the population resorted to what the author calls "marginal activities", including the theft of state resources, trafficking in all kinds of goods on the black market, private activity with or without a licence, satisfying the needs of foreign tourists, and even prostitution and robbery. According to Bloch, the authorities would have tolerated – to a certain extent – these activities, as long as citizens refrained from expressing political criticism and participated in mobilizations organized by the authorities.

Such remarks are undeniably relevant, but popular adherence to the socialist regime – as the author himself acknowledges – can also be explained by the influence of "the utopia that presents the Cuban Revolution as the embodiment of a people in permanent struggle against the enemies, external and internal", who are trying to destroy it.³⁴ Over time, this idea has evolved into considering "unanimity and homogeneity its core values" and has made of any alternative to the current political system "a threat to be combated". This is how the norms, values and principles promoted by the national leadership's political discourse – reproduced in school textbooks and repeated ad nauseam in the press – have managed to impose themselves on the collective imagination, leaving little room for other ways of conceiving the history and even the future of the Cuban nation.

In short, the fact that Cuba has become throughout its revolutionary period a country without a tradition of anti-government demonstrations or popular uprisings, for the many reasons mentioned above, is precisely what makes it possible to highlight the exceptional nature of the events that took place there on July 11, 2021. Although the latter failed to become a sufficiently broad and unifying social outburst capable of

---

[33] It should also be noted that several hundred thousand Cubans have sought a solution to their problems by migrating to other countries, especially the United States, throughout the revolutionary period. Many of them with the capacity to oppose the island's regime left, in the process, a huge void in the national protest arena.

[34] The author points out that such statements and some very common expressions usually used in media and official discourse – such as "treason" or "conspiracy in the service of a foreign power" – might not be completely devoid of political relevance, given the close ties that internal dissidence has always maintained with officials of the US Interests Section in Havana or its proven funding by US government agencies. See: Bloch, Vincent (2009), "Reflexiones sobre la disidencia cubana", in *Análisis político*, 67, 91.

bringing about immediate changes in the political regime in place since 1959, it must be acknowledged that these events constitute a clear break in the recent history of the Caribbean island.

Cuba's 11J in the global context resulting from the pandemic

We have just examined some of the factors that contributed to making 11J an atypical case within the Latin American protest arena and an extraordinary event in the history of revolutionary Cuba. If the events of that day were to be framed in the global context in which they took place, it would be difficult to ignore the close links they have with the social dynamics observed at the same time in different parts of the world. Let us elaborate briefly on this last point.

In numerous countries the coronavirus health crisis was accompanied by an increase in protest demonstrations by their citizens – regardless of their size, political system, macroeconomic situation or how their respective governments responded to the crisis. According to information from the Armed Conflict Location and Event Data Project compiled by Zachariah Mampilly[35] – professor of international relations at the Marxe School of Public and International Affairs at New York University – between 2019 and 2020 the number of demonstrations worldwide increased by seven per cent despite the confinements, and other provisions aimed at limiting public gatherings, adopted at the time by political and health authorities. As Mampilly points out, the objectives of demonstrators in poor or developing countries certainly differed from those of protesters in rich countries: in general, the former demanded greater and faster access to vaccines against the Covid-19 virus as well as more help to stay afloat economically, while the latter demanded the relaxation of certain government measures that sought to mitigate the effects of the pandemic but were perceived as restrictions on their civil rights and liberties. Beyond this fundamental difference, however, they all had at least one thing in common: they were the expression of a social dissatisfaction – which had been brewing for some time – with

---

[35] Mampilly, Zachariah, "Citizens Have Had Enough", *The New York Times*, October 12, 2021.

the inability of the ruling classes to serve and protect the majority of their populations, especially the middle and lower classes.

The origin of this popular discontent and the low level of trust placed in political elites at the time varied, of course, from case to case. For most countries with democratic regimes, Mampilly traces it back to the 2008 financial crisis. According to him, this crisis highlighted the shortcomings of "the social contract imposed after the Cold War between governments and their peoples" – a contract that "was largely based on the idea that market-centred policies would lead to prosperity and peace in the world". In the case of many Latin American and Caribbean nations that have also been rocked recently by an unprecedented cycle of protests, the despair of millions of citizens and their mistrust for their respective governments may stem from even more complex socio-economic and political processes. As political scientist María Victoria Murillo (Murillo 2021: 6–7) – Director of the Institute of Latin American Studies at Columbia University, New York – explains, beyond the specific characteristics of each country, there are two main reasons for this situation: first, the slowdown in economic growth since the early 2000s, with the consequent implementation of budgetary adjustments by national governments and the interruption of the trend towards a reduction in poverty and inequality rates that large sectors of society had enjoyed until then. Second, the numerous cases of corruption that have been uncovered in various parts of the region, reinforcing the conviction of many citizens that political and economic elites collude to maximize their own profits and neglect basic concerns of the vast majority of the population. Finally, with regard to Cuba – as we saw earlier – the growing citizen dissatisfaction revealed by the protests and riots of 11J can largely be explained by the acute crisis the country had been experiencing and whose dire consequences for the well-being and quality of life of the population had only worsened, despite attempts to reform the economic system undertaken by the Cuban government at the beginning of 2021.

Whatever the primary causes of the discontent that led almost simultaneously to millions of people demonstrating – peacefully or violently – in streets and squares around the world, what was at stake across the board was the serious crisis of representation and trust that had been undermining relations between peoples and their rulers for quite some time. Within this context, the deteriorating health, economic and social situation resulting from the Covid-19 pandemic was the last straw, exacerbating pre-existing inequalities within society and overturning the social safety nets on which the most vulnerable depended then and still depend today. Logically, this led to greater dissatisfaction and distrust among citizens regarding the ability of their leaders and public institutions to find solutions to their most pressing problems, igniting – or rekindling – the flame of protest in many corners of the globe. The pandemic would thus have acted as an aggravating factor in an already highly complex situation. These were precisely the circumstances that were identified as a crucial element to help us understand what happened in Cuba on July 11, 2021.

The impact of the coronavirus in Latin America and the Caribbean, although much more serious than what was experienced in Cuba, is another telling example of the above. It is true that the wave – or rather, "the tide"[36] – of citizen protests that had been flooding Latin American and Caribbean streets and squares with some regularity began months before the onset of the health crisis, and was particularly powerful during the second half of 2019. In fact, between July and November of that year alone, popular demonstrations took place in Chile, Colombia, Panama, Peru, Honduras, Haiti, Puerto Rico, Venezuela, Nicaragua, Ecuador and Bolivia. It is also true that with the outbreak of the pandemic, and after the first restrictions on internal movement came into force, the number of protests dropped significantly. In the course of 2020, however, new hotspots of conflict and tension emerged and others that seemed to have been extinguished were reactivated – some of them even spreading throughout the following year. It is clear that the Covid-19 crisis then played a key role in the outburst of social unrest at the regional level. It is therefore worthwhile to dwell briefly on this last factor.

For the countries of Latin America and the Caribbean, the arrival of the coronavirus crisis posed an unprecedented multidimensional challenge, starting naturally with the health dimension. As reflected in a report by the Economic Commission for Latin America and the Caribbean (ECLAC 2022b: 100–106), prior to this crisis the health systems in the area had already major structural weaknesses, lacking sufficient resources and capacity to provide access to quality services to the poorest and most disadvantaged groups in society. Moreover, living conditions in many Latin American cities were – and still are – not optimal. As social science

---

[36] See: Vázquez Zamora, Juan, "Descontento social y protestas en América Latina: ¿ola o marea?", *El País*, November 13, 2019.

researcher María Mercedes Di Virgilio (Di Virgilio 2021: 77–78) points out, "a very large part of the region's population [...] lives in slums or informal neighbourhoods, [...] does not have access to decent housing and [...] therefore lacks drinking water for personal hygiene". All this would considerably limit the positive impact of the prevention measures initially implemented to control the transmission of the virus there. Thus, despite the increase in critical hospital capacities – intensive care unit beds, staff, ventilators, etc. – health systems found themselves in a situation of overflow and even collapse, especially from the first half of 2021.[37]

On the other hand, although with important differences from one nation to another, access to vaccines against the coronavirus was extremely slow. By the end of 2021, in more than half of the Latin American and Caribbean countries, less than 50 % of the population was fully vaccinated (ECLAC 2022b: 22). As a direct consequence of all of the above, the number of infections increased exponentially and the human toll was devastating – a situation that, moreover, did not allow for any improvement in the near future. In fact, Latin America and the Caribbean had "the highest number of deaths reported by COVID-19 in the world (1,562,845 up to December 31, 2021), a figure that will unfortunately continue to grow as long as the pandemic persists. These represent 28.8 per cent of all reported COVID-19 deaths worldwide, despite the fact that the region's population is only 8.4 per cent of the world's population" (ECLAC 2022b: 17). It is clear, then, that the region was totally unprepared to face such challenges, with even more dramatic consequences for its inhabitants.

The same lack of preparedness and equally serious repercussions were also to be deplored in the economic dimension. In the years prior to the pandemic, growth in most countries in the region was close to zero, due to low levels of investment and productivity in their economies, among other reasons, as well as high levels of informal employment and unemployment. These structural deficiencies would become even more

---

[37] As in the case of Cuba, this was mainly due to the emergence of variants of the virus that were characterized by greater transmissibility and caused more severe disease, a significant decrease in antibody protection, a reduction in the effectiveness of treatments and vaccines, or even failures in the diagnosis of the virus. See on this topic: ECLAC (2022b), *Panorama Social de América Latina, 2021*, Santiago de Chile, 18.

noticeable after the sharp slowdown in activity throughout 2020, durably hampering economic development. In fact, as the ECLAC itself warned (2022a: 61), the gradual relaxation that year of the measures enacted to contain and mitigate the pandemic allowed for an effective increase in the dynamism of activity and, incidentally, a certain recovery in most macroeconomic indices. However, that recovery was not sufficiently robust, so GDP levels remained below those recorded in the period prior to the health crisis.

The impact on the labour market was particularly significant, with a prolonged decline in employment and labour participation – 30 % of jobs lost in 2020 were not recovered in 2021 – which essentially affected the most vulnerable population groups. For example, the greatest difficulties in re-entering the labour market were observed among the least educated group of working women, who were also the most affected by job losses during the first year of the pandemic (ECLAC 2022a: 14). The impact was equally uneven according to the age of the workers; it was worse among young people who not only had to bear the negative effects on their education and training but also faced significant obstacles when looking for a first job or changing jobs. According to data for the year 2020 (ECLAC 2022b: 16), "the unemployment rate of young people was twice as high as that of adults and reached 23 % on average, equivalent to 7 million people between 15 and 24 years of age". Finally, the same asymmetric trends were registered in terms of the recovery of employment by occupational category, with those of lower quality being the fastest to recover. In fact, as ECLAC points out again (2022a: 82), "self-employed workers, most of whom are informal, had a faster rate of employment recovery than wage earners". Precisely, the relative growth in employment recorded in 2021 was mainly due to the rise in informal sector employment. This, while generally an improvement over the previous year's situation, was not entirely satisfactory, as it meant that many Latin American and Caribbean households would earn incomes that were still insufficient to alleviate the hardship caused by the coronavirus. Consider also that these households, being part of the informal sector, lack access to social protection and unemployment insurance benefits. In sum, it is clear that one of the most pernicious effects of the deterioration of the economic situation generated by Covid-19 was the increase in job insecurity and even more unequal access to the labour market in most countries of the region.

Finally, it was no surprise that – in addition to deepening pre-existing economic and social gaps – the worsening health and economic situation also led to an increase in the levels of poverty and extreme poverty of a large part of the population. The estimates published by the Economic Commission for Latin America and the Caribbean (2022b: 14) leave no doubt in this regard: "In 2021, the extreme poverty rate have reached 13.8 per cent and the poverty rate would go as high as 32.1 per cent. Therefore, compared to 2020, the number of people in extreme poverty would increase from 81 million to 86 million, while the total number of people in poverty would slightly decrease from 204 million to 201 million. […] the estimated relative and absolute levels of poverty and extreme poverty have remained above those recorded in 2019".

Another element that undoubtedly contributed to prolonging the social crisis that these data reflect was the change, of course, taken in 2021 in terms of fiscal policy. Specifically, this involved the suspension – or reduction – of certain emergency measures implemented in 2020 to support families and protect the productive structure.[38] Public spending had been one of the main fiscal instruments used, with a significant increase in subsidies and transfers aimed at alleviating the effects of the pandemic on household and business incomes. This increase, carried out in a context marked by a reduction in tax revenues, logically translated into an expansion of fiscal deficits and a substantial increase in public debt in many countries in the region. The reaction of several national governments in the course of 2021 was therefore to try to reduce these deficits and stabilize the debt by withdrawing or reducing the fiscal impulse of the previous year. Unsurprisingly, this shift in priorities primarily affected the most vulnerable layers of society.

In short, the seriousness of the health, economic and social situation in Latin America and the Caribbean since 2020 has become evident. This situation and the ruling classes' inability to manage it were certainly additional reasons for dissatisfaction for millions of citizens, further widening the popular rejection of the national political leaders and institutions, which in turn led to a new cycle of protest in several countries in the region. This illustrates very well what happened almost simultaneously

---

[38] The fiscal packages implemented after the outbreak of the pandemic were unprecedented in scope and represented on average 4.6 % of the region's GDP. See: ECLAC (2022a), *Balance Preliminar de las Economías de América Latina y el Caribe*, Santiago de Chile, 89.

in many parts of the world. We believe that the events in Cuba are fully in line with this global dynamic. Of course, it cannot be denied that the latter occurred in less serious circumstances than those observed in other corners of the planet, especially in its closest geographical environment. As previously explained, compared to other nations in the region, such events had also a less far-reaching impact and scope. Even so, it is difficult to interpret the reaction of the thousands of Cubans who took to the streets that day as anything other than deep resentment for the prolonged crisis they had to face and their rulers' inability to find quick and effective solutions to it. It is precisely at this point that the main convergences between the events of 11J and the rest of the demonstrations that took place worldwide at the time are to be found.

Conclusions

Having analysed and put into perspective the events occurred on July 11, 2021, in several Cuban cities we come to the conclusion that – although unprecedented and with their own particularities – they are not unique or an isolated case within the global context of mass protests resulting from the pandemic crisis. It does not mean, of course, that the significance of the situation that led to such events should be underestimated or ignored. The fact that for the first time in its history the country's political authority is challenged by a small but significant part of its population demonstrates the extent to which the impact of this crisis has been detrimental to the life and well-being of the Cuban people nationwide. It is also indicative of the destabilizing effect of the crisis that it was the first time as well that the island did not remain on the sidelines of a wave of popular protests that began in other parts of the world.

One year after 11J, a great deal of uncertainty prevails in this country. On the one hand, it seems clear that the most critical moments of the pandemic have been overcome. At the time of writing, health authorities were reporting an average of only 67 infections per day,[39] 0 deaths and 321 active confirmed cases still in hospital. The massive use of three Cuban vaccines had already been authorized, and 9,976,437 people, 90 % of the population, were reported to be fully vaccinated (MINSAP

---

[39] According to data published on the website of the Ministry of Public Health of the Republic of Cuba (MINSAP), between July 17 and 19, 2022.

2022). The state also seems determined to strengthen its control mechanisms over civil society. According to *Cubalex*, a Cuban human rights NGO,[40] legal instruments have been passed in recent months that make it even more difficult to exercise freedom of expression on the internet. Another cause for concern is the new Penal Code, which includes "criminal offences against State Security that criminalise citizen participation in matters of public interest, with long sentences that can lead to life imprisonment and the death penalty". Finally, it is difficult to perceive – despite this NGO's statements to that effect – the awakening of citizen awareness and the strengthening of civil society organizations that could serve as catalysts to rapidly mobilize broad sectors of the population and promote a real social outburst. On the other hand, however, popular unrest is still very palpable today. The problems related to shortages of food, medicines and other basic necessities, as well as constant power cuts, which led thousands of Cubans to take to the streets a year ago, not only remain unresolved but have worsened even further. The impression is that the slightest incident can shatter the current tense and fragile calm. It remains impossible though to predict the course the island might take over the medium and long term.

Bibliography

Alonso Sánchez, Jorge (2020). "Movimientos populares y la pandemia del Covid-19" in *América Latina después del 2020*, Roncal Vattuone, Ximena, and Robinson Salazar Pérez (coord.), Buenos Aires, Elaleph.com, 21–66.

Bloch, Vincent (2009). "Reflections on Cuban dissidence", in *Political Analysis*, 67, 83–104.

Comisión Económica para América Latina y el Caribe, ECLAC (2022a), *Balance Preliminar de las Economías de América Latina y el Caribe. 2021*, Santiago de Chile.

——— (2022b). *Panorama Social de América Latina. 2021*, Santiago de Chile.

Del Castillo, Siro (2014). "Una visión de la crisis de los balseros en el XX aniversario", paper presented at the symposium "Recordando la crisis

---

[40] Morfi, Giselle, "A un año del 11J: ¿Qué pasó ese día? ¿Qué ocurrió después?", *Cubalex*, July 3, 2022.

de los balseros y sus consecuencias, 20 años después", Cuban Research Institute at Florida International University.

Dirección de Registros Médicos y Estadísticas de Salud del Ministerio de Salud Pública de Cuba (2021), *Anuario Estadístico de Salud*. 2020, Havana.

Di Virgilio, María Mercedes (2021). "Desigualdades, hábitat y vivienda en América Latina", in *Nueva Sociedad*, 293, 77–92.

Geoffray, Marie Laure (2012). *Contester à Cuba*, Paris: Editions Dalloz, 2012.

International Crisis Group (2021). "Paro y pandemia: las respuestas a las protestas masivas en Colombia", in *Latin America Report*, 90, p.43.

Mesa-Lago, Carmelo (2021). "Las causas de las protestas y la magnitud de la crisis económica en Cuba", in *Horizonte Cubano*, https://horizontecubano.law.columbia.edu/news/las-causas-de-las-protestas

Ministerio de Salud Pública. República de Cuba, MINSAP (2022). "Coronavirus en Cuba. Información oficial del MINSAP", Havana.

Murillo, María Victoria (2021). "Protestas, descontento y democracia en América Latina", in *Nueva Sociedad*, 294.

Oficina Nacional de Estadísticas e Información de la República de Cuba, ONEI (2022), *Anuario Estadístico de Cuba*. 2021, Havana.

Oxfam International (2016). "New dynamics of communication, organisation and social action in Latin America. Technopolitical reconfigurations", https://www.oxfam.org/es/informes/nuevas-dinamicas-de-comunicacion-organizacion-y-accion-social-en-america-latina.

Solar Cabrales and Frank Josué (2021). "La frustración del odio", in *Miradas en contexto. Aproximaciones desde la universidad a la Cuba actual*, González Santamaría, Abel Enrique (ed.), New York: Ocean Sur, 12–15.

Epilogue: Intersectional solidarity and fairness in Ibero-American counteractions

MARINA RUIZ CANO (Le Mans Université)

Health crises are due to many reasons, as different chapters in this book have demonstrated. Nowadays we tend to think immediately about viruses or medical issues, but the truth is that natural, political and social contexts are factors that generate health crises, and therefore elements that need to be analysed. At the same time, these areas also serve to address health problems, looking for causes, responsibilities and solutions. Take, for example, the impact of toxic discharges into water, which seep into the phreatic table and directly affect food. This is another area where a responsible policy that respects the health of the population should be developed. Many health problems are due to poor or low-quality nutrition, and the situation is aggravated by the many additives in ready-made meals, including several addictive ingredients, which are at the root of chronic diseases such as diabetes. Of course, the issue of food cannot be separated from the conditions of production, in particular the use of chemicals and GMOs. We cannot forget the scandals surrounding Round-up, and we must not overlook the disastrous consequences of the current policy of Monsanto, whose GM seeds provoke bioethical and economic problems – think of the privatisation of the market with the banning of certain types of seeds and varieties. The high meat consumption and the fact that the majority of agricultural land is used for the production of animal products also have an impact on the availability of food for the entire world population, which is already eight billion. This figure is expected to reach 10 billion by 2025, so the percentage of starving people will continue to rise if no action is taken.

Another sector at risk is nuclear energy, which has been strongly contested by several social movements. Faced with the climate emergency, other sectors are focusing their struggle not only on human health but also on the health of the Earth, with its flora and fauna, in order to prevent the ecocide underway, particularly visible in Latin America. Let us cite just a few examples of the attacks on nature perpetrated in 2021: an oil spill extinguished the aquatic life of rivers and streams in Guatemala, hundreds of trees were felled in Colombia to build an electricity grid, as well as several specimens of *Bulnesia sarmientoi* trees in Paraguay – which was also an attack against autochthonous culture – the Chilean ecosystem of the Estero Lircay wetland was destroyed to promote a property project and 18 million bees died of poisoning in Costa Rica due to the use of agrochemicals.

Women usually lead struggles against ecocides, especially in Latin America. Ecofeminism becomes a movement that clearly seeks to care for others, starting with nature, and to confront the ferocious patriarchal capitalism that undermines the health of the population, whether through miserable working conditions, which also cause illness and even death, or through industrial pollution or the destruction of the environment. The main victims of neoliberal logics are the precarious people, women and minorities, whose precariousness pushes them, for example, to buy cheaper and poorer quality food, which has a negative impact on their health. The food shortages they face have led to recent looting of supermarkets and food shops not only in Cuba but also in Spain in August 2012, when unemployed people and trade unionists took more than 3,000 kilos of staple foods as a form of protest. At the same time, these vulnerable sectors suffer the most psychologically, and the Covid-19 pandemic has exacerbated, and at the same time brought to light, the psychological health problems of Western societies. Loneliness appears as a cause of distress and the consumption of antidepressants and other drugs linked to psychological problems is on the rise, especially among the younger generations. This means that pharmaceutical companies are making profits at the expense of the population's health. This theme inspired, for instance, Antonio Altarriba's Spanish graphic novel *Yo, loco* (2019). The dichotomy that establishes the opposition between health and economics is precisely the driving idea of several works in this volume.

The destructive effects of economic policies on public health have been alerting the population for years. If we take the case of Spain, and more specifically the Community of Madrid, citizen protests have been organised since 2012 in a collective called "Marea Blanca" (White Tide). This movement, which is part of the social dynamics initiated by the 15-M movement, is demonstrating against the closure of numerous health centres and the acceleration of health privatisation. The management of the current government of Isabel Díaz Ayuso is plunging Madrid's public health system into a deep crisis, massively contested in a demonstration

Epilogue - Solidarity in Ibero-American counteractions

on 13 November 2022, which, according to government figures, brought together 200,000 people in the capital – 678,000 according to the organisers. It is worth remembering that article 43 of the Spanish Constitution "recognises the right to health protection" and states "it is the responsibility of the public authorities to organise and protect public health through preventive measures and the necessary benefits and services".

If the crisis has been used to impose strict social control measures – imposing full vaccination for access to leisure, transport or even work – the media have also played an important role in the consolidation of emotional communities facing the pandemic. At the same time, they have been at the service of governments to transmit the directives of the expert cabinets. Such discourses have not been free of a certain technocratic manipulation, as analysed in one of the articles, with a specific vocabulary that aims to guide social actions and interactions. Another problematic aspect lies in the confusion of the principles of veracity and verisimilitude – fiction and reality, therefore – which leads to state interference or intervention in everyday life by dubiously ethical means. This reality calls into question the possibility of thinking about health policy, leaving political and electoral interests aside.

It is worth noting that digital communication has taken root as a political strategy. In turn, it is the ground where current protests are taking place. In this sense, an analysis of the role of opposition parties, for example, in Uruguay or Spain, offers clues about the political instrumentalisation of the crisis as a weapon to criticise the present government. The management of the population's uncertainty, a large part of which was constantly consulting the news for information – with more than alarming news, by the way – has led to an "infodemic", that is, an excess of information on the Covid-19 pandemic. Argentina's Ministry of Culture warned in April 2021 about its dangers, in particular because this "overabundance of information online or in other formats" includes "deliberate attempts to spread false information". In a statement, the World Health Organisation (WHO) said, "Misinformation and misinformation can harm people's physical and mental health, increase stigmatisation, threaten health gains and encourage non-compliance with public health measures, reducing their effectiveness and jeopardising the ability of countries to curb the pandemic."

The war of images, whose sensationalism is used as a tool for political and discursive manipulation, must also be analysed and contested. The staging or theatricalisation of illness or mourning has a major emotive capacity that raises the ethical problem of the representation of the sick and dying. This taste for the abject, to use Julia Kristeva's expression, reinforces the power of horror and undermines human dignity. The press occupies a fundamental place here, feeding, or not, social attitudes of protest or conformism. A detailed and qualitative analysis of pandemic and war discourse by country therefore seems essential to restore human dignity and to expose political shortcomings in the economic, health, social and educational fields. This last area has been the scene of numerous measures that go against learning and equality. We can think of the digital divide and its consequences – as well as constituting a violation of the right to privacy and private life, with the leaking of personal data in Chile through the platforms used by schools, governed by capitalism and the principle of constant surveillance. This consolidates the rupture of the separation between the public sphere (work) and the private sphere (home).

The outbreak of criticism of the management of the pandemic has led to a rise of the extreme right in several countries, which claims the role of leader of social protest, as if its anti-system proposals were the key to effectively helping society. Once again, we find a paradigmatic case of this usurpation in Madrid, where there were several demonstrations against confinement and against health security or prevention measures. This denialism derives largely from the force of a neoliberal ideology that extols the individual and economic profit, to the detriment of the common good. In this respect, the Spanish coalition government formed by PSOE and Unidas Podemos does not offer an exemplary model either, as it instrumentalised not the economic crisis but the Basque left-wing pro-independence party EH Bildu in May 2020. The extension of the state of alarm – a situation declared by the Council of Ministers in the face of public catastrophes or health crises that allows extraordinary measures to be taken – needed support. EH Bildu made its approval possible in exchange for fully repealing the labour reform of the previous PP government and improving the living conditions of Spanish workers. A few hours after the extension of the state of alarm, the government backtracked on the signed agreement and limited the modifications in labour matters, showing once again that collective interests do not always take precedence over electioneering, pressure from the opposition, good press or the economic benefits of a minority.

Another factor that explains the impulse of more than dubious discourses of the extreme right has to do with the new meanings given to the term "freedom", as shown by the protest slogans with the management of

Epilogue - Solidarity in Ibero-American counteractions 225

the pandemic in Uruguay ("Freedom or death") or Madrid ("Freedom or socialism"). Protestant and liberal sectors have wanted to appropriate the principle of freedom that, according to their speeches, is actually nothing more than a defence of individualism and consumption. Moreover, these discourses do not hesitate to question the impartiality of science, which, although it should be questioned in a constructive way, should in no way be used to underpin neoliberal policies. The supremacy of these capitalist logics is also reflected in the solidarity funds imposed on civil servants, but not on the private sectors. The unfair or unequal distribution of health resources has been a source of controversy in Spain for years, and the presence of foreign retirees who come to Spain for surgery and to take advantage of the 100 % public health system of the Spanish state, which does not exist in their countries of origin, is a source of indignation. A certain left-wing melancholy emerges that sees the social protests provoked by the recent health crises as a failure. Although the origin of the situation is to be found in capitalism, the consequence is that this political and economic system has once again emerged strengthened, as shown by the profits of big business, the supremacy of Amazon, gentrification or the inflation of basic health products and of the shopping basket before the energy crisis broke out.

As for tourism, it is clear that this sector has been hit hard by the health crisis, causing closures, redundancies and astronomical economic losses. As one of Spain's economic engines, this crisis has led to several ERTE (Expediente de Regulación Temporal de Empleo), which are nothing more than temporary collective redundancies due to lack of activity or income. In this case, the State has proposed some economic measures to help those affected, but it is necessary to consider the double-edged nature of these ERTEs, since they sometimes serve as a pretext for employers to do away with part of their employees. The problem, in the context of the Covid pandemic, is that collective social mobilisations were not allowed in the first place, and the fear of the disease has considerably weakened the strength of the demonstrations. The paradigm shift in the discourses on the pandemic has produced a rupture in the strategies of contestation, which seems to inaugurate a new, more naïve era, whose excessive reliance on digital communication and science anaesthetises protest movements. In this sense, it is worth noting that these protests show generational differences.

Paradoxically, tourism is a sector that also benefits from the harmful consequences of climate change, which will ultimately accentuate health and survival problems. An example of this is the rise of drought tourism in Spain, which consists of visiting completely dry and empty water reservoirs that reveal the ruins of past buildings, which hints at an imminent national crisis of water resources, the basis for agriculture, i.e. food, and above all for life.

We have mentioned the sectors that are most vulnerable to the crisis, but we would like to insist in particular on the situation of women, which has not been addressed in the various articles in this volume. Women occupy the majority of care professions in hospitals, nursing homes, schools and supermarkets. Not only are they on the front line but their pay is also not commensurate with what they offer to society. Added to this injustice is the growing insecurity on the streets after confinement, to the extent that some women have claimed that the mask offers them protection because it makes them invisible – a contradictory statement to say the least, as the veil is often criticised. It would therefore seem that this invisibilisation was desired by certain sectors of women's society. In any case, this reality highlights a problem of citizen security in many cities, at the origin of several citizen mobilisations in Spain and Latin America – think of the strength of 8 March – but to which governments have not yet come up with effective responses. The situation is all the more worrying given the proliferation of voices raised against the right to abortion – which is finally making progress in Latin America, albeit slowly, after the decriminalisation of abortion in Argentina and Colombia.

Women's right to control their own bodies is also a public health issue, and policies are needed to guarantee access to contraceptives and terminations of pregnancy. Otherwise, women risk their lives by having clandestine abortions, again resorted to by the poorest women. Challenges to these women's health rights should be seen as protests to prevent health crises, both physical and psychological. The same is true for other sectors that are demonised in many societies: LGTBIQ+ groups or sex workers. The risks range from psychological illnesses, which can lead to drug use, to diseases such as hepatitis or AIDS, which can also be considered pandemics. Finally, one should not forget the situation in prisons, where prisoners often live together in poor hygiene and security conditions – the struggle of the prisoners' union COPEL in Spain during the 1970s is an example of the protests provoked in these places. In addition, drugs have been used in prisons as a weapon to anaesthetise these outcasts of society, as well as other dissident groups.

Epilogue - Solidarity in Ibero-American counteractions

Against this backdrop, where society is driven by the value of money and the exploitation of the weakest, effective solutions are needed. Health crises could be avoided by policies that respect the environment, by an equitable distribution of the planet's goods and wealth, or by dismantling the economic system as it is currently conceived. Indeed, the obsession with productivity is at the root of accidents that kill thousands of workers every year and leads to chronic physical and psychological illnesses. Stress, depression and burnout are other 21st-century pandemics against which we should raise our voices. Perhaps an ecofeminist approach, based on respect for life and for others, considered our equals, is a strategy to follow. It is not surprising that women, especially in Latin America, lead more and more protests. Similarly, the key to dealing with crises of any kind, including health crises because of the economic, political and social consequences they entail, is solidarity and trade union, family and class support.

However, these solidarity networks, which appear, for example, in communal gardens or urban farms, have their limits. In some cases, this supposed solidarity is nothing but false philanthropy – think of the case of Inditex owner Amancio Ortega and his donations of medical equipment when he evades taxes. Close to this eagerness to profit from everything does José Luis Martínez Almeida, who strangely enough opted for one of the most expensive offers, as evidenced by the mask business of Luis Medina and Alberto Luceño, who sold gold-priced masks to the Madrid city council, lead corruption. On the other hand, the population performs functions that should be provided by the government, thus highlighting the tension between state and community.

Finally, artistic creation is also a way of dealing with the problems arising from health crises. On the one hand, dissent voices that want to restructure the current fragmented society find their place in art. The word clearly has a subversive power that is symptomatic of the state of health of any democracy: the more numerous the conflicts, the better the health of the democratic system, since freedom of expression implies dissent. Illness is also a creative engine, and fever functions as an artificial paradise that makes it possible to escape from an increasingly cruel world, plagued by traumatic silences. Art is thus a form of resistance and contestation capable of confronting any crisis and inventing alternative worlds that will not necessarily find a massive echo in the digital media but will mature in the shadows, discreetly, silently. That is where all its subversive capacity lies.

www.ingramcontent.com/pod-product-compliance
Ingram Content Group UK Ltd.
Pitfield, Milton Keynes, MK11 3LW, UK
UKHW021838140426
5217IPUK00022B/1509